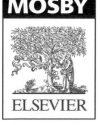

Flesh and Bones of
MEDICAL
MICROBIOLOGY

Andrea Guyot FRCPath MSc Dr Med DTM&H DipHIC
Consultant Microbiologist
Frimley Park Hospital, Frimley, UK

Silke Schelenz FRCPath PhD MSc Dr Med DipHIC
Clinical Senior Lecturer and Consultant Microbiologist
Norfolk and Norwich University Hospital, Norwich, UK

Steven Myint MD MRCP Dr rer nat DipClin Micro
Visiting Professor of Medicine and Microbiology
University of Surrey, Guildford, UK

Illustrations by Jennifer Rose

MOSBY

ELSEVIER

Edinburgh   London   New York   Oxford   Philadelphia   St Louis   Sydney   Toronto   2011

MOSBY
ELSEVIER

First published 2010

ISBN 978-0-7234-3382-8

British Library Cataloguing in Publication Data
A catalogue record for this book is available from the British Library

Library of Congress Cataloging in Publication Data
A catalog record for this book is available from the Library of Congress

Notice
Knowledge and best practice in this field are constantly changing. As new research and experience broaden our understanding, changes in research methods, professional practices, or medical treatment may become necessary.

Practitioners and researchers must always rely on their own experience and knowledge in evaluating and using any information, methods, compounds, or experiments described herein. In using such information or methods they should be mindful of their own safety and the safety of others, including parties for whom they have a professional responsibility.

With respect to any drug or pharmaceutical products identified, readers are advised to check the most current information provided (i) on procedures featured or (ii) by the manufacturer of each product to be administered, to verify the recommended dose or formula, the method and duration of administration, and contraindications. It is the responsibility of practitioners, relying on their own experience and knowledge of their patients, to make diagnoses, to determine dosages and the best treatment for each individual patient, and to take all appropriate safety precautions.

To the fullest extent of the law, neither the Publisher nor the authors, contributors, or editors, assume any liability for any injury and /or damage to persons or property as a matter of products liability, negligence or otherwise, or from any use or operation of any methods, products, instructions, or ideas contained in the material herein.

Printed in China

The
publisher's
policy is to use
**paper manufactured
from sustainable forests**

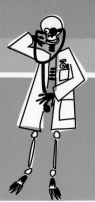

Contents

The big picture

Medical microbiology in its broad scope of covering both laboratory and medical aspects of infection is a topic that is important in all branches of medicine. Worldwide, there are more people affected by microbial disease than all the other diseases combined and the differential diagnosis of every non-infectious disease (other than purely surgical diseases) includes infection. The rapid evolution of microbes also means that this is a disease area that does not remain static, and new infections are being recognized every year. It is also important to note that not only the diseases but also the microbes themselves need to be understood as, despite a large number of anti-microbial agents, these diseases continue to cause significant morbidity and mortality. Some of this is from classic infectious disease but these agents are also known to cause diseases such as gastric ulcer and thought increasingly to be causal factors in conditions such as ischemic heart disease and cancer.

The study of medical microbiology is the examination of a balance between the host, humans, and a very large army of potential invaders. These invaders share one unique feature, that of being very small, with most either invisible or near invisible to the naked eye. Those of medical importance are not only the ones that cause disease but also those that are beneficial to humans. The latter group include the **commensals**, those organisms that 'naturally' inhabit our non-sterile body spaces and surfaces, and the **probiotic bacteria**, which are increasingly added to boost natural defences against pathogenic, disease-causing microorganisms.

Medical microbiology is subdivided into four main study areas:

- **virology**, the study of the smallest type of microorganism, the viruses
- **bacteriology**, the study of the type of agent for which we have the most available therapies, bacteria
- **mycology**, the study of fungi, which are generally environmental contaminants that can cause damage if they get into sterile body spaces
- **parasitology**, the study of the largest microorganisms, the protozoa and medical worms (helminths).

Microorganisms have been noted since the 17th century, with the Dutchman Anton van Leuwenhoek being attributed as writing the first description of microbes in a letter to the Royal Society of London in 1674. Until the mid-19th century, however, these 'microbes' were thought to arise spontaneously from non-living matter. In 1861, Louis Pasteur, a French chemist, first argued that these were organisms that existed in the environment and grew as living things. The German physician Robert Koch subsequently developed the germ theory of disease, which stated that these organisms were also responsible for illness. Since then, we have identified several hundred infectious agents and specific therapies for a fraction of these. Infectious diseases worldwide are the most common cause of illness.

Host–parasite balance

There is a fine balance between the host and the pathogen: the 'home' and away' teams (Fig. 1.1). Pivotal in this balance is the normal human microflora, which is present on both external and internal body surfaces. The adult human body is estimated to contain 10^{13} cells but there are 10^{14} microorganisms that colonize it. These 'normal' flora can be divided into two groups: the resident flora (Fig. 1.2), which are present continually, and transient flora, which may be there for weeks. These are part of the 'home' team in that they compete antagonistically for nutrients (and other resources) with potential pathogens. Infection occurs when either these organisms invade body spaces which are normally sterile or a pathogenic organism gains a foothold. Infection does not always lead to injury, but when it does the term 'infectious disease' is used. When infectious disease is transmissible from person to person, it is termed communicable. Infection with the human immunodeficiency virus (HIV), leading to the acquired immunodeficiency syndrome (AIDS), would be a

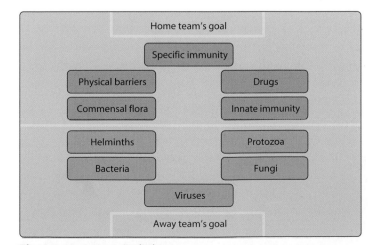

Fig. 1.1 Host–parasite balance.

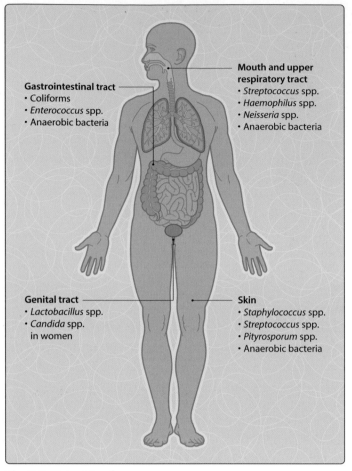

Gastrointestinal tract
• Coliforms
• *Enterococcus* spp.
• Anaerobic bacteria

Mouth and upper respiratory tract
• *Streptococcus* spp.
• *Haemophilus* spp.
• *Neisseria* spp.
• Anaerobic bacteria

Genital tract
• *Lactobacillus* spp.
• *Candida* spp. in women

Skin
• *Staphylococcus* spp.
• *Streptococcus* spp.
• *Pityrosporum* spp.
• Anaerobic bacteria

Fig. 1.2 Colonizing flora.

good example of a communicable disease, whereas tetanus is usually caused by soil contamination of a wound and not passed from person to person.

Pathogenesis

There are two main mechanisms of host damage by microorganisms (Fig. 1.3): direct injury and damage by toxins. Direct injury occurs from those that are invasive and destroy tissue by taking over normal cellular processes (viruses tend to take this route), multiplying and occupying space (most bacteria) or by removing essential nutrients. The second mechanism by which invading organisms can cause damage is through being, or producing, toxins (chemical poisons) that harm host cellular machinery.

Broadly speaking, there are some key stages in pathogenesis.

Adherence or attachment to host cells. The mechanism whereby this occurs may also contribute to an infection being specific to an organ or system if there is a specific interaction with a host macromolecule.

Invasion. This may be by direct growth or aided by the presence of virulence factors, such as hyaluronidases and proteases, which enhance tissue breakdown.

Systemic spread. Bacteraemia and septicaemia occur when bacteria have invaded superficial tissues and enter the bloodstream, thus enabling them to gain access to distant sites.

Damage by toxins. These molecules are produced by living organisms and are capable of causing disease on contact with, or absorption by, body tissues. Toxins vary greatly in their effects, ranging from usually minor and acute (e.g. bee sting) to almost immediately deadly (e.g. botulinum toxin). There are two types of toxin produced by bacteria:

■ exotoxins: soluble proteins released into the surrounding environment
■ endotoxins: part of the cell membrane but are still 'poisonous'.

Bacterial exotoxins are some of the most potent cellular 'poisons' known: 1 ng botulinum toxin is sufficient to be lethal to a guinea pig or human. They are often subclassified on their site of action: **enterotoxins** affect the gut, **neurotoxins** affect the nervous system and **cytotoxins** have general cellular toxicity. Endotoxin is the lipopolysaccharide component of the outer membrane of Gram-negative bacteria.

Once a pathogenic sequence is commenced, then the **host response** will affect its severity and timespan. Both innate and acquired immune reactions are important in combating infections.

Clinical features of infection

An infection typically goes through a number of stages as it causes disease (Fig. 1.4). Initially, there may not be any obvious clinical symptoms: this is the incubation period. The microorganism is still multiplying but the body reaction is insufficient for it to be noticed clinically. Then there is often a prodrome, where there are some non-specific symptoms, that is, the individual 'is not quite right' but there are no defining features. These then lead to specific symptoms. At this time, the host immune response is maximal and actually contributes to the symptomatology. If the infection is naturally controlled by the host defence mechanisms, then there is a resolution or decline period followed by convalescence, where the patient is able to resume normal activities of daily living and then complete recovery.

Diagnosis

The diagnosis of infection can theoretically occur at any of these clinical stages. Except when there is an outbreak of disease, however, it is unlikely that diagnosis will be attempted in the incubation period. After this period, the ideal is to be able to detect the pathogen directly: this can be achieved by direct sight (microscopy, electron microscopy or by the naked eye), culture or by gene detection. An alternative is to detect the specific immune response to the infection, IgM antibody early in infection or IgG after 10–14 days.

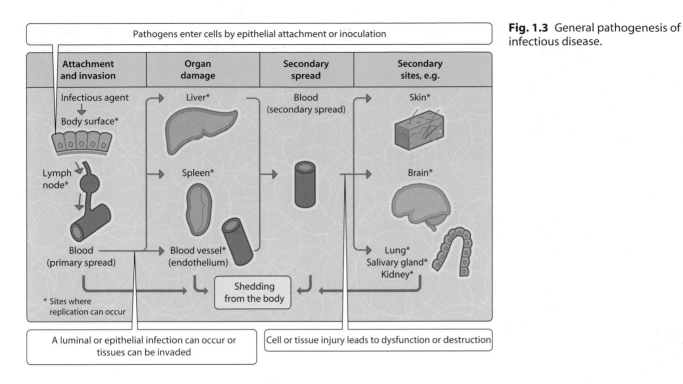

Fig. 1.3 General pathogenesis of infectious disease.

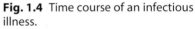

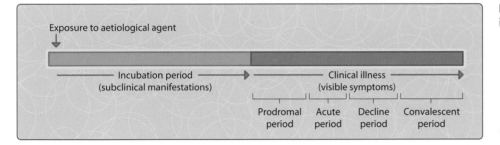

Fig. 1.4 Time course of an infectious illness.

Treatment and prevention

Not all infections resolve spontaneously and some require specific interventions. There are antimicrobial drugs available for all the major types of microorganism: antibiotics for bacterial infections are the most commonly used, but antiviral, antiprotozoal, antifungal and anthelminthic compounds are all available. The principle of all these agents is that they target a specific part of the physiology or life cycle of the pathogen that is not present, or is less important, in the host. With antibacterial agents, this has been relatively easy as prokaryotic cells are structurally and functionally distinct from the eukaryotic cells of humans. Viruses use host cell mechanisms and protozoa and helminths are eukaryotes, so for these it is harder to create a drug with specificity of action; consequently, the drugs often have greater toxicity for the host.

The principles of **public health** are to prevent infection and the spread of infection through control of the environment. Arguably the control of the environment, through water sanitation and other processes that clean the external world, has had the most impact on infection control. Prevention through **vaccination** has had the second biggest impact but **infection control measures**, where isolation and hygiene are key, have the greatest impact on individuals rather than populations.

High-return facts

1 There are four main types of microorganism that cause infectious disease: viruses, bacteria, fungi and protozoa. Bacteria are prokaryotes whereas fungi and protozoa are eukaryotes. Prokaryotes do not have a nucleus, whereas eukayotes do.

2 Viruses contain either DNA or RNA but not both and may or may not have an envelope. The capsid, or shell, can have one of three basic morphologies: icosahedral, helical and complex. Viruses can cause cell lysis, may replicate without destroying the cell or may enter a latent phase with little or no replication.

3 All bacteria have a lipid bilayer cytoplasmic membrane, which is coated with peptidoglycan to provide mechanical stability. In Gram-positive bacteria, the peptidoglycan layer is thick, whereas in Gram-negative bacteria it is thin and overlaid by an outer membrane. The outer membrane controls the movement of substrates into the cell. Some bacteria possess immunologically important polysaccharide capsules or fimbriae and some a flagella for movement. Some bacteria require specialized staining or detection techniques (e.g. *Mycobacteria* require a Ziehl–Neelsen stain). Most bacteria multiply by binary fission within 20 min. They contain a circular chromosome and extrachromosomal DNA on plasmids.

4 Fungi are eukaryotic organisms; the medically important species are the yeasts (unicellular organisms), moulds (filamentous fungi) and dimorphic fungi (moulds that transform into yeasts at body temperature). Fungal infections (mycosis) can be superficial, subcutaneous or invasive and disseminated. Serious infections are often caused by opportunistic fungi (e.g. *Aspergillus*) that do not normally cause infection unless a person is immunosuppressed.

5 Protozoa consist of a single eukaryotic cell. They reproduce either asexually by binary fission or sexually. The commonest are the amoebae, flagellates and the ciliates. Many are harmless but some cause serious disease, particularly in areas of socioeconomic deprivation and in the immunocompromised.

6 Parasitic helminths comprise the nematodes (roundworms), cestodes (tapeworms) and trematodes (flukes). They most commonly cause gastrointestinal and visceral infections. As with the protozoa, infections are difficult to treat because of the lack of agents that are specific for the infective organism.

7 Human transmissible degenerative encephalopathy is caused by prions. The commonest is Creutzfeldt–Jakob disease (CJD), which is characterized by a spongiform degeneration of the brain. This has a long incubation period followed by progressive cognitive impairment, ataxia, myoclonus and extrapyramidal signs. Variant CJD affects younger patients, is more rapidly progressive and is linked to eating meat from cows infected with bovine spongiform encephalopathy (BSE).

8 Prevalence is the number of cases of infection per unit of population at a single point in time. Incidence is the number of new cases per unit of population over a specified time period. Infections are considered in public health terms based on their spread: outbreaks, epidemics, pandemics.

9 Koch's postulates are a means of confirming that an infectious agent is the cause of a disease. Classically they can be stated as (a) the organism occurs in every case of the disease and under circumstances which account for the pathological changes and clinical course of the disease; (b) the organism occurs in no other disease as a fortuitous and non-pathogenic finding; (c) after being isolated from the body and grown in pure culture, the organism will repeatedly produce the same clinical disease when inoculated into a new susceptible host; and (d) the organism can then be isolated from the new host.

10 The pathology caused by an infectious agent can be the result of direct damage by the infectious agent (e.g. cell death) or can result from the host's immune reaction to that agent, immunopathology. There are four types of immunopathological reaction, mediated by different mechanisms. Infection by some viruses is linked to cancer causation.

11 Innate host defences to infection comprise physical barriers (such as skin), commensal bacteria, local environment (such as pH and mucus), secreted enzymes (such as lysozyme) and phagocytic cells.

12 The adaptive host responses can be classified broadly into those that involve B cells and those that involve T cells. B cells produce antibodies of which here are five classes: IgA, IgG, IgM, IgD and IgE. Foreign antigens are recognized by T helper cells, which produce a range of cytokines and these determine the nature of the immune response.

13 The distinction between influenza illness and common cold can be made clinically based on the former having an abrupt onset, high fever and greater constitutional upset. Bacterial infections of the upper respiratory tract can be secondary to a viral infection. While some infections are self-limiting, others require acute medical intervention, such as diphtheria and epiglottitis.

14 Respiratory viruses (e.g. influenza, parainfluenza, adenovirus) induce tracheobronchitis, which can become superinfected by bacteria (e.g. *Staphylococcus aureus* and *Haemophilus influenzae*). Respiratory syncytial virus causes bronchiolitis in infants and pneumonitis in the immunocompromised. Pneumonia is typically caused by *Streptococcus pneumonia*e and its therapy is guided by severity assessment. Therapy ranges from home therapy with amoxicillin to broad-spectrum antibiotics and ventilation. Mycoplasmas cause atypical pneumonia, characterized by lung consolidation and a non-productive cough. Legionellae are transmitted by droplets dispersed from stagnant water (fountains, air conditioners) and cause severe pneumonias in the immunosuppressed.

15 Mycobacteria are a group of thin, rod-shaped bacteria that require special staining (e.g. Ziehl–Neelson stain) for detection. The most common infections in humans are tuberculosis (caused by *M. tuberculosis*) and leprosy (caused by *M. leprae*). Classic clinical features of pulmonary tuberculosis are low-grade fever, night sweats, weight loss and productive blood-stained cough. Leprosy may present as lepromatous leprosy in patients with a poor immune response. They have multiple skin lesions packed with mycobacteria, causing nerve damage and deformation of extremities. Patients with a good cell-mediated response may develop tuberculoid leprosy, which is characterized by fewer skin lesions containing few or no mycobacteria.

16 Viral meningitis, which is characterized by a lymphocytic cell predominance in cerebrospinal fluid (CSF), is commonly caused by herpes simplex virus, enterovirus and the mumps virus. Meningococcal sepsis affects mainly infants and teenagers and is responsible for half the cases of bacterial meningitis; it is characterized by a neutrophilic cell predominance and high protein in the CSF. In countries where vaccination against meningococcus C has been introduced, meningococcal meningitis has become rarer, and it is mainly caused by meningococcus B in western Europe. Pneumococcal meningitis occurs in asplenic or otherwise immunosuppressed patients and requires early treatment with β-lactams and steroids to prevent neurological sequelae.

17 Encephalitis and brain abscess affect the brain itself; myelitis affects the spinal cord, and neuritis or polyneuritis affects nerves. Infection of nervous tissue often leads to long-term sequelae. Infections occur in the brain either through direct inoculation in trauma or by the infection crossing the blood–brain barrier. Encephalitis is predominantly a viral disease whereas brain abscesses are predominantly bacterial in origin or caused by zoonoses. Neuritis/polyneuritis occurs from direct infection of nerves. Some infections produce neurotoxins, which interfere with synaptic transmission.

18 The eye has a number of external structures that can get infected such as the eyelid (blepharitis), sebaceous glands (stye), the cornea (conjunctivitis) and the surrounding soft tissue (orbital cellulitis). Pathogens may be introduced from the environment (fungi, *Pseudomonas*) or the skin (*Staphylococcus aureus*) following accidental trauma, surgery or contaminated contact lenses, causing exogenous infection of the eye. Infections may progress to the back (posterior) part of the eye (vitreous humour, retina and choroid) causing endophthalmitis and potential loss of vision. Such infection can also occur after a bloodstream infection (endogenous route) but this is much rarer.

19 Viral skin rashes predominantly occur in childhood and have four basic components: maculopapules, vesicopustules, papulonodules and haemorrhages. These can occur either on a mucous membrane, an enanthem, or on the cutaneous surface, an exanthema.

20 The skin is made up of several different layers (epidermis, dermis and subcutis) all of which can be infected. Superficial infection of the epidermis can be caused by bacteria (impetigo) or fungi (ringworm/dematophyte infections). Infections of hair follicles may lead to folliculitis. Boils (furuncles or carbuncle) are result from infection of follicles and sebaceous glands. Many of these skin infections are caused by *Staphylococcus aureus* or *Streptococcus pyogenes*. Uncontrolled spread of bacteria into the dermis can lead to cellulitis (red, hot skin and fever) or life-threatening necrotizing fasciitis of deeper tissues. Some organisms release gas (*Clostridium* spp.) when introduced deep into damaged tissue, causing gas gangrene.

21 All areas of the gastrointestinal tract can be targeted by infecting microorganisms. *Helicobacter pylori* infection is associated with gastritis and peptic ulcers. Bacteria (e.g. *Campylobacter* and *Salmonella* spp.) in undercooked food or viruses (e.g. norovirus) cause gastroenteritis, which presents as vomiting, diarrhoea and abdominal discomfort. *Salmonella typhi* spreads by the faecal–oral route. Colitis is characterized by abdominal cramps and haemorrhagic diarrhoea (dysentery) and can be caused by *Shigella* spp. in tropical countries or by verotoxin-producing *Escherichia coli* (VTEC); VTEC can also lead to the haemolytic uraemic syndrome. In hospitals, *Clostridium difficile* affects elderly patients taking antibiotics, and symptoms range from diarrhoea to pseudomembraneous colitis with toxic megacolon. Food poisoning is caused by preformed bacterial toxins in food and is characterized by a short incubation period of a few hours.

22 Viral hepatitis has the classic triad of jaundice, dark urine and pale stools. There are five main types of hepatitis virus, A–E, of which B, C and D are transmitted by blood and bodily secretions whereas A and E are transmitted faecal–orally. Hepatitis can also be caused by bacterial and amoebic infections. Liver abscess can be caused either by primary infection or by secondary spread; peritonititis can follow contamination of the peritoneal cavity. The biliary tract and pancreas can become infected following obstruction to their drainage.

23 Bacterial endocarditis affects patients with valvular abnormalities leading to regurgitations (audible murmur). Intermittent bacteraemias with viridans streptococci, enterococci or staphylococci can cause adhesion of the fibrin–platelet nidus to predamaged valves. Patients present with fever of unknown origin and the diagnosis is based on echocardiographic evidence of a vegetation and a persistent bacteraemia. Antibiotic therapy for 4–6 weeks and, in severe cases, valve replacement are required for cure. Infection of heart muscle (myocarditis) is usually viral and pericarditis requires drainage.

24 Women are more at risk of urinary tract infections (UTI) because they have a shorter urethra. Children and men with recurrent UTIs should be investigated for anatomical anomalies in the urinary tract. Uncomplicated UTI (cystitis in women) needs to be distinguished from pyelonephritis, the latter requiring longer antibiotic therapy and frequently leading to bacteraemia. UTI is characterized by pyuria and bacteriuria. Asymptomatic bacteriuria (in the absence of pyuria) is significant if repeatedly demonstrated in pregnancy and infancy. Coliforms are the most common isolates. UTI is difficult to diagnose by urinalysis and culture in patients with an indwelling urinary catheter and remains a clinical diagnosis.

25 Chlamydia and genital warts are endemic among those 16–24 years of age. Urethritis is nowadays more commonly caused by chlamydia than *Neisseria gonorrhoeae*. Chlamydia can lead to ascending infections in the genital tract, presenting as pelvic inflammatory disease or prostatitis. Herpes simplex virus causes a relapsing painful vesicular rash on the genitals, which requires treatment with aciclovir. Genital ulcers can be a manifestation of syphilis, lymphogranuloma venereum, chancroid or granuloma inguinale. Vaginal discharge caused by candida or bacterial vaginosis is not a sexually transmitted disease but rather a disturbance of normal vaginal flora.

26 Congenital intrauterine infections comprise toxoplasmosis, rubella, cytomegalovirus and herpes simplex virus (TORCH), to which should be added *Trepenoma pallidum* (syphilis), varicella zoster virus (German measles) and parvovirus. The last does not cause malformations, but fetal bone marrow suppression can lead to hydrops fetalis. Intrauterine infections can be diagnosed by demonstrating maternal seroconversion during pregnancy or by polymerase chain reaction examination of amniotic fluid at 20 weeks of gestation or of blood from the newborn. Perinatal infections derive from infectious agents in the birth canal. Group B streptococci are transmitted after rupture of membranes and cause sepsis and meningitis in the neonate. *Chlamydia trachomatis* and *Neisseria gonorrhoeae* can cause ophthalmia neonatorum. Neonatal hepatitis B infections can be prevented by hepatitis B vaccination after birth. HIV transmission can be prevented by peripartum antiretroviral therapy and the avoidance of situations where vertical transmission can occur: caesarian section rather than natural birth and omission of breast feeding.

27 Bone infection (osteomyelitis) occurs if bacteraemia settles in haematomas near growth plates of long bones in children, in intervertebral discs or in prosthetic joints. Exogenous infections of bones are common in deep foot ulcers or in open fractures. Magnetic resonance imaging is more sensitive than radiograph for the diagnosis. Osteomyelitis requires antibiotic treatment for 4–6 weeks and infected prosthetic joints often require revision arthroplasty. Joint infection (septic arthritis) follows haematogenous spread and needs a joint washout and 3–6 weeks of antibiotic therapy. Reactive arthritis is caused by an immune response to infectious agents such as *Chlamydia trachomatis*, particularly in patients carrying *HLA-B27*. Bacterial infections of muscle can progress to gangrene.

28 Septicaemia is characterized by the presence of bacteria in the bloodstream (bacteraemia) combined with physical signs such as fever, tachycardia and hypotension. There are a number of Gram-positive (e.g. *Staphylococcus aureus*) and Gram-negative (*Echerichia coli*, meningococcus) bacteria that commonly cause this condition, which should be treated with antibiotics.

29 HIV is a retrovirus, meaning that it must first convert its RNA into DNA before it can reproduce within infected cells. HIV can be transmitted sexually; through blood products; through injecting drug use, and accidental needlestick injuries; and from mother to child. HIV infects T lymphocytes and macrophages; when the immune system begins to fail, AIDS-defining illnesses, often opportunistic infections, commence. Treatment with a mixture of antiretroviral drugs can slow the progression of the infection but there is no cure such as a vaccine at present.

30 Immunosuppressed patients are particularly susceptible to infections and become vulnerable to opportunistic infection by normally harmless organisms. Risk groups include those with a primary congenital defect in the immune system and those with secondary immunodeficiency through HIV infection, chemotherapy, alcoholism or diseases such as diabetes mellitus. T cell suppression as seen in HIV infection or organ transplantation may cause reactivation of viruses (cytomegalovirus, herpes simplex virus) and intracellular pathogens are more difficult to control (*Salmonella*, *Listeria*). A low neutrophil count (neutropenia) renders patients vulnerable to invasive fungal infections (e.g. aspergillosis) and serious bacterial sepsis.

31 Zoonoses are infections transmitted from reservoirs in animals. The animals may be asymptomatic. Common zoonoses are Lyme disease and campylobacter. Newly emerging infections frequently have their reservoir in animals, such as avian influenza or West Nile virus in birds. Zoonoses can cause fever, skin rashes and/or meningoencephalitis.

32 Fever, diarrhoea, respiratory tract and skin infections are common in the returning traveller from tropical countries. Infections with enteropathogenic *Escherichia coli*, *Giardia lamblia*, salmonella, campylobacter and cryptosporidium present as gastroenteritis, whereas *Entamoeba histolytica* and shigella infections present as dysentery (colitis). Giardiasis and amoebiasis require therapy with metronidazole. Besides malaria, dengue fever and viral hepatitis are common causes of fever in the traveller. Tropical skin infections comprise furuncles, trapped maggots (myasis, tungiasis), migrating hookworm (larva migrans) and cutaneous leishmaniasis. Travel clinics offer vaccination and advice on prevention.

33 Malaria is an infection by the protozoan *Plasmodium* spp. that is spread by the bite of an infected female *Anopheles* mosquito. It is a major health problem facing the world. *P. falciparum*, *P. malaria* and *P.ovale* are common in the tropics, whereas *P. vivax* can also occur in subtropical climates. *P. falciparum* causes severe parasitaemia, leading to complications of cerebral malaria and hypoglycaemia. Quinine and artemisinin derivates are preferred for the treatment of falciparum infections. *P. vivax* and *P. ovale* can form liver hypnozoites, which induce relapses. Non-falciparum malaria remains susceptible to chloroquine.

34 Soil-transmitted nematodes like *Enterobius vermicularis*, *Ascaris*, hookworms, whipworms and strongyloides have a complex life cycle: after their eggs have been swallowed, their larvae migrate through the lung before the adult worms settle in the bowels. *Strongyloides* and hookworms can survive in soil and infect humans by penetrating the skin. Tapeworms are acquired by eating undercooked meat, which contains cysticerci, and the adult worms grow from the small bowel to the rectum, where they shed proglottides. *Echinococcus* is a tapeworm of dogs and foxes. In humans, the larvae get trapped in the liver capillaries and form a hydatid cyst. Schistosoma eggs are excreted in human faeces and urine and after a complex life cycle in lakes form cercariae, which penetrate the skin of swimmers. They reach the portal vein and deposit eggs in bladder and rectum, causing chronic inflammation.

35 Pyrexia of unknown origin (PUO) is defined as an illness with fever >38.3°C for more than 3 weeks in duration and no specific diagnosis after 1 week of investigations. In the immunocompetent host, infections, neoplasms (e.g. lymphomas), collagen vascular diseases and drug fevers are possible causes. A number of common infections present as PUO. Diagnosis requires radiological imaging, serological tests for Epstein–Barr virus, cytomegalovirus and *Coxiella bunettii* and eventually biopsies of lymph nodes, skin or liver.

36 Increased international air travel, change in the environment, globalization of food supplies and breakdowns in public health services have lead to the emergence and spread of new (e.g. severe acute respiratory syndrome) and re-emerging (e.g. tuberculosis) infectious diseases. Raised awareness, surveillance, improved diagnostic tests and treatments are important to control and contain these diseases.

37 The principle of hospital infection control is to prevent and control hospital-acquired (nosocomial) infections. This can be achieved by minimizing exposure to microorganisms (e.g. decontamination of equipment), controlling the route of transmission of infectious agents (airborne, faecal–oral or contact) by placing an infected patient in isolation (e.g. carrier of methicillin-resistant *Staphylococcus aureus*) and by promoting good hand hygiene.

Infections may also be prevented by treating underlying diseases (e.g. diabetes) and using antibiotics rationally and effectively (e.g. good antibiotic policies, surgical prophylaxis).

38 The hospital environment and medical devices (e.g. surgical instruments) have to be safe for patients and staff. Depending on the type of device, the risk of infection can be low (skin contact only, e.g. washbowl), intermediate (contact with mucous membranes, e.g. bronchoscope) or high (contact with sterile body sites, e.g. surgical instruments). Cleaning, disinfection and/or sterilization depending on the risk are, therefore, important to prevent contamination and transmission of infections.

39 Microbial contamination of food and water can lead to a number of infections. The most common food poisoning bacteria are *Salmonella* and *Campylobacter* spp., which can cause diarrhoea after consumption of contaminated food such as undercooked chicken. Faecal contamination of drinking water or recreational water can also pose a health risk. Poorly maintained air-conditioning systems, spars or showers can cause air-borne infections such as legionnaire's disease. Good sanitation, safe drinking water and maintenance of air-conditioning units, showers and baths are important measures for the prevention of such infections.

40 Antibacterial agents inhibit bacterial growth by interfering specifically with a function of a bacterial cell that is not present in the host cell. Resistance is when bacterial growth cannot be inhibited by achievable serum concentrations. Some bacteria are intrinsically resistant (chromosomal gene) to certain antimicrobial drugs, whereas most bacteria develop resistance by acquisition of mobile gene elements (e.g. transposons, plasmids) or by mutation. Antibiotic choice is determined by the likely microorganisms, the pharmacokinetics to reach the infected site, drug safety and, lastly, costs.

41 Antibacterial agents can be classified by their mode of action and by their range of activity against different bacterial species, broad- and narrow-spectrum antibiotics. Dosing regimens must consider choosing the right drug, getting the drug to the target site (absorption, distribution) and maintaining sufficient drug concentrations (drug metabolism and excretion) for a sufficient length of time. For some drugs, the margin between therapeutic and potentially toxic concentrations, the therapeutic index, is small and plasma drug concentrations may need monitoring (e.g. gentamicin).

42 Antiviral agents target the specific life cycle of the virus. Broadly this will be virus attachment, entry, uncoating, transcription, translation, packaging and egress. Most currently available antiviral agents target transcription/translation. Antiviral drugs are available for herpesvirus, influenza, hepatitis and HIV. The drug regimens for HIV are complex to reduce the risk of developing resistance.

43 The treatment of fungal infections depends mainly on the causative fungus, the site and the severity of the infection. Superficial dermatophyte infections may just be treated with topical agents (e.g. terbinafine) whereas invasive fungal infections (e.g. *Aspergillus*) require systemic treatment. Antifungal drugs act through disruption of the cell membrane or inhibition of cell wall or protein synthesis. Not every antifungal agent will be effective against all fungal species.

44 Choice of antimalarial agent depends on the species of *Plasmodium*, the occurrence of drug resistance and whether prophylaxis or therapy is intended. Agents with activity against *P. falciparum* comprise quinine, artemisins and mefloquine. For prophylaxis, atavoquone with proguanil can be used in areas endemic with *P. falciparum*. Metronidazole and tinidazole are active against intestinal protozoa (*Giardia lamblia*, *Trichomonas vaginalis* and trophozoites of *Entamoeba histolytica*). For the eradication of *E. histolytica* cysts, diloxanide furoate is necessary. Nitazoxanide has activities against most protozoa, even *Cryptosporidium parvum*, helminths and anaerobic bacteria. Ivermectin paralyses nematodes and is mainly used for onchocerciasis. Albendazole achieves good tissue concentrations and is used for tissue stages of helminths, larva migrans and echinococci. Mebendazole is poorly absorbed and is effective only for intestinal stages of helminths. Praziquantel paralyses tapeworms and flukes and is the drug of choice for schistosomiasis.

45 Immunization is a public health measure to prevent infectious diseases. Active immunization involves the administration of a specific immunogenic substance (vaccine) to induce a protective antibody response by the person's own immune system (e.g. hepatitis B vaccine). Passive immunization produces immediate immunity by giving ready-made antibodies from a pool of immune blood donors (e.g. tetanus hyperimmune immunoglobulin serum). Patients without a (functional) spleen are particularly susceptible to infections caused by encapsulated bacteria (*Haemophilus influenzae*, *Staphylococcus pneumoniae* and *Neisseria meningitidis*) and certain parasites (e.g. malaria). Antibiotic prophylaxis may be given to prevent infections.

46 Most of the time the oral cavity contains a microflora of bacteria, fungi and viruses living in a fine balance and without causing disease. Food debris attached to teeth supports the growth of mouth bacteria, forming dental plaque in which the bacteria exist in a biofilm system that is protected from antimicrobial action. Tooth decay and gum disease can occur. Oral bacteria can also enter the bloodstream if trauma occurs in the mouth (poor hygiene or dental treatment). Normally this is a transient bacteraemia but it can cause endocarditis in the vulnerable (e.g. with prosthetic heart valves or immunosuppressed).

Fleshed out

Microorganisms can be divided into prions, viruses, bacteria, fungi and parasites. All but prions contain nucleic acids, whereas prions are non-degradable host proteins that can be transmitted in the food chain or by tissues. Chapters 1–7 characterize the different infectious agents.

Microorganisms are ubiquitous in the environment and normal human flora. However, pathogenic infectious agents invade tissues and cause direct cell damage or immune-mediated inflammation. The pathology of inflammation is described in Chapters 8–12; Chapter 35 widens the pathogenesis to non-infectious causes for fever when discussing pyrexia of unknown origin.

Infection can affect almost every human organ and Chapters 13–28 describe the organ-specific manifestations from skin to brain. Chapter 46 on oral microbiology complements this textbook.

Certain infectious agents only affect the immunocompromised host (Chs 29 and 30) or are specific for certain environments (Chs 31–34), for example malaria depends on the Anopheles mosquito as vector, or are zoonoses (Ch. 31) and require contact with the animal that harbours the infection.

Since the middle of the last century, antimicrobial drugs have been available and have reduced the morbidity and mortality associated with infections. Chapters 40–44 give details on antimicrobial therapy for bacterial, viral, fungal and helminthic infections. However the incidence of infections had been decreasing before the introduction of antimicrobial agents. This was achieved by improving hygiene (e.g. clean water supplies), sterilization of instruments and infection control in hospital environments (hand hygiene), all of which reduced the transmission of pathogens. Chapters 37–39 describe the methods available for sterilization, disinfection and food and water hygiene. Immunization (Ch. 45) against infectious diseases renders the potential hosts non-susceptible to infectious agents. Successful vaccines have been developed for endemic infections with high morbidity or mortality, such as meningococcus group C, pneumococcus and measles.

1. Introduction to microorganisms

Questions
- What are the features of eukaryotes and prokaryotes?
- What are the features of the principal classes of micro-organism?

Microorganisms are mostly harmless and **non-pathogenic** (non-disease causing), and indeed may be beneficial. It is estimated that a human body carries approximately 10^{14} cells, but only 10% of these are human in origin; the rest is microbial flora. There is not a consensus definition of a microbe but broadly speaking they are organisms which are not visible to the naked eye. Medical microbiology is the study of microscopic organisms and their effect on humans. Traditionally, slightly larger organisms that cause infectious disease, such as helminths, are usually included and this book will keep to that tradition. It encompasses their biology, diagnosis, treatment and prevention.

If morbidity and mortality from infection is to be reduced, a number of issues must be considered. The environment must be managed through public health measures to reduce the chances of contact with virulent microorganisms. In hospitals, this process is called 'infection control' and it includes steps to ensure that patients with hazardous agents do not disseminate them to others. Innate and specific immunity are clearly important in determining the outcome of contact with pathogenic organisms; we must understand how immunity works, what happens when it is disturbed through modern medical treatments and how it might be increased by methods such as immunization. Disease must be diagnosed quickly and accurately, either clinically or through laboratory methods, before it has spread to others or the individual is too ill to be saved. We must develop and apply high-quality, evidence-based treatments which include the prompt and appropriate use of drugs; the ideal antibiotic will kill the infecting microorganism but not the commensal bacterial flora or the patient, and yet will not lead to antibiotic resistance amongst virulent bacteria over time. Infections are extremely common, and it is vital that all medical doctors thoroughly understand basic microbiology if they are to prevent, diagnose and treat infections effectively.

Prokaryotes and eukaryotes

There is a vast array of agents that are capable of causing human disease (Fig. 3.1.1). A 'family tree' of all living organisms is shown in Fig. 3.1.2. This tree, with its three main branches, is very different from that suggested in the 1980s and has come about because

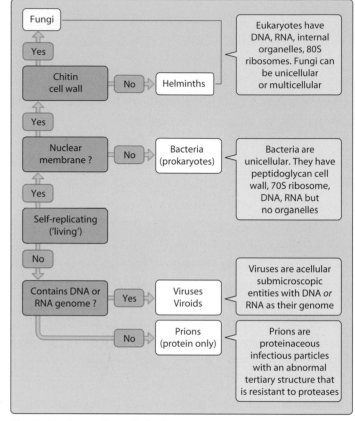

Fig. 3.1.1 Properties of infectious agents.

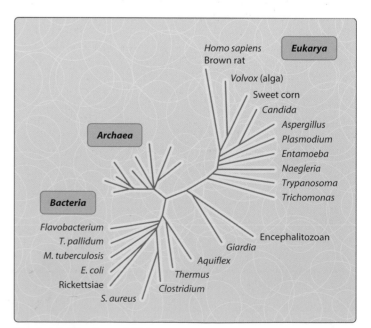

Fig. 3.1.2 The 'tree of life'.

of advances in molecular biology. The eukaryotic domain is a single group with almost unbelievable diversity, from single-celled amoebae through worms, fungi and plants right up to complex animals such as humans.

The prokaryotes are divided up into two fundamentally separate domains: the Archaea and Bacteria. But just because many bacteria look the same under the microscope, it does not follow that they will behave similarly—indeed there is as much difference between the genes of the bacteria *Treponema pallidum* and *Staphylococcus aureus* as there is between those of humans and sweet corn! The relative sizes of these organisms are shown in Fig. 3.1.3.

Archaea. The Archaea are a group of prokaryotes that live in extreme conditions such as thermal pools. While they may be very important to the health of natural environments, they are not known to cause human infection.

Bacteria. These are very significant when it comes to human health, both because some of them must live on us or in us if we are to remain healthy (our **commensal** flora) and because some of them are capable of causing disease.

Eukarya. This group has larger, more diverse and complicated cells and includes fungi (yeasts and moulds) and parasites (single-celled protozoa and helminths).

Viruses, viroids and prions. These are not truly 'living' agents but are transmissible and able to replicate.

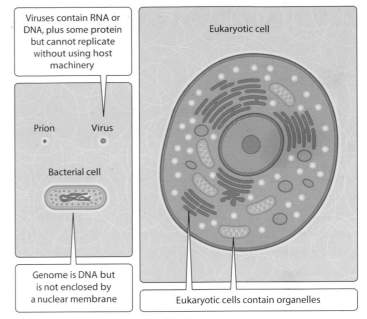

Fig. 3.1.3 Relative sizes of infectious agents.

CASE STUDY: Manifestations of infection

AB, a 22-year-old Trinidadian, presented to the dermatologist with a nodular skin rash. It was mildly pruritic, erythematous and although widespread was mainly on the trunk. It had been present for 3 months and was becoming progressively nodular. He is domiciled in the UK but had recently returned from a visit to Trinidad. He complained of tiredness. Physical examination showed a temperature of 37.8°C and axillary and inguinal lymphadenopathy. His initial full blood count and biochemistry was normal apart from a raised serum calcium and mild lympho cytosis.

A blood film was made to detect malarial parasites but was negative. The film did show numerous abnormal white cells. Subsequent skin biopsy showed a deep perivascular infiltrate of lymphocytes and a bone marrow trephine showed erythroid and megakaryocytic hyperplasia. Serology for human T cell lymphotropic virus type 1 (HTLV-1) serology was positive, confirming a diagnosis of adult T-cell leukaemia lymphoma (ATLL) caused by HTLV-1 infection. He was treated with chemotherapy

This case has many lessons, but the most important one is that infectious disease can manifest as non-infectious disease and needs to be in the differential diagnosis of most presenting conditions. It also illustrates that, across the globe, regional epidemiology needs to be taken into account. Although ATLL is uncommon in HTLV-1 infection, when it occurs it tends to be in those of African, Caribbean or Japanese origin.

2. Viruses: the basic facts

Questions
- What are the basic properties of viruses?
- How are viruses classified?
- How do viruses replicate?

Viruses are named from the Latin for poison (venenum). They are the smallest and simplest of replicative agents of infection in humans. They are both the commonest organisms found in nature and the most frequent cause of human infection. The following properties distinguish them from living (prokaryotic and eukaryotic) cells:

- they are acellular and have a simple organization
- they possess *either* DNA or RNA in the same structure
- they cannot replicate independently of host cells.

Viruses can exist extracellularly, as **virions** with few, if any, enzymes, and intracellularly, when they 'hijack' the host biochemical machinery to produce copies of virion components.

Virions are 15–400 nm in diameter and exhibit one of five basic morphologies (Figs 3.2.1 and 3.2.2). They basically consist of a shell, called a **capsid**, which may be icosahedral or helical in shape. Capsids may be surrounded by an outer membrane, called the **envelope**. There is a further structure type, termed complex, with a capsid structure that is neither helical nor icosahedral; these complex viruses may also possess an envelope. The capsid is an arrangement of protein subunits, termed protomers or capsomeres. Enclosed within the capsid is the genetic material, which is either RNA or DNA, and may be single or double stranded. If single-stranded RNA, this may be capable of acting as messenger RNA (mRNA), so-called **positive sense**, or it will have to be made into a complementary copy to do so, termed **negative sense**. Some genomes are also segmented, such as rotaviruses.

Viruses produce acute, persistent or chronic and latent infections. In latent infections, the virus is dormant for long periods and may not produce detectable virions. Apart from the classic diseases, viruses are increasingly recognized as causes of cancer (e.g. hepatoma) and autoimmune disorders. It should also be noted that there are many 'orphan' viruses, such as adeno-associated viruses and hepatitis G virus, for which a disease has yet to be established.

Classification of viruses

Viruses are currently classified into different taxonomic groups on the basis of:

- the nature of the host (animal, plant, bacterial, insect or fungal)

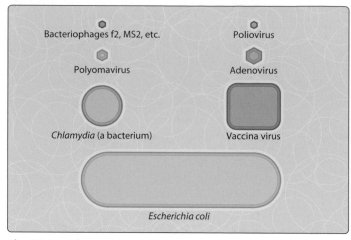

Fig. 3.2.1 Relative sizes of viruses.

- whether they possess an envelope
- the type of nucleic acid they possess
- the morphology of their capsid
- the diameter of the virion or nucleocapsid
- their immunological properties
- the intracellular location of viral replication
- their clinical features, i.e. disease(s) caused and method of transmission.

The first three of these are the most commonly used. In addition, there is a commonly used term 'arbovirus', which encompasses a range of virus families which are all *ar*thropod *bo*rne. The term 'phage' is used to denote viruses which parasitize bacteria (i.e. **bacteriophage**).

The most commonly used simple classification is the Baltimore classification, which is based on their genome and mode of replication (Fig. 3.2.3).

Viral replication

All viruses make copies of themselves in the intracellular phase. The major difference between viruses is their strategy for genome replication. All viruses have to generate mRNA to produce protein and nucleic acid copies.

The end result of viral infection may be

- lysis of the cell
- lysogeny where the host cell is not destroyed but continues to support viral replication
- latency where there is little, or no, viral replication.

In the last two states, the viral genome may be integrated into that of the host.

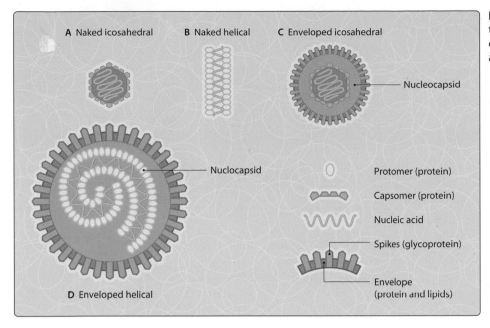

Fig. 3.2.2 Basic virus morphology. In addition to the four forms shown here, there is complex morphology that does not follow a regular structure.

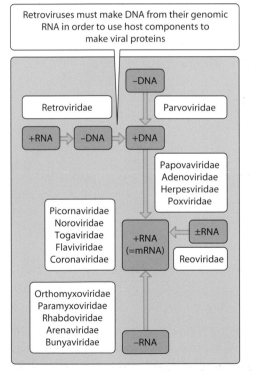

Fig. 3.2.3 Baltimore system of classification of viruses. +, coding strand; −, negative sense; ±, two complimentary strands.

Viral replication is not perfect, and mutant genomes are also made: this is the means by which viruses evolve. Non-replicative mutants are termed **defective-interfering** (DI) particles, which interfere with the replication of the initial virus.

3. Bacteria: the basic facts

Questions
- Which cell structure differs between Gram-negative and Gram-positive bacteria?
- Which structure is used for conjugation?

Bacteria are divided into two main groups on the basis of chemical staining (with the Gram stain) and light microscopy: Gram positive and Gram negative. The differential staining is based on a major difference in the cell wall (Fig. 3.3.1). Both have a lipid bilayer **cytoplasmic membrane** with various inserted proteins, the most important of which are membrane-spanning **permeases**. These control active transport of nutrients and waste products in and out of the cell. A complex web of cross-linked **peptidoglycan** outside the cytoplasmic membrane provides the cell with mechanical strength. It is particularly abundant in Gram-positive organisms, when it also contains strands of **teichoic** and **lipoteichoic acid**. Gram-negative organisms have an additional **outer membrane** enclosing a thin layer of peptidoglycan and enzymes within the **periplasm**, an environment controlled by the movement of substrates through membrane **porins**. Some bacterial species may have a loosely adherent **polysaccharide capsule** exterior to the cell wall and possibly additional structures which project from the cell surface (Fig. 3.3.2):

- **flagellae**: whip-like cords, typically 0.02 μm thick, 10 μm in length; cells move by rotating the flagellae
- **fimbriae** (**pili**): hair-like structures typically 6 nm thick, 1 μm long; they carry **adhesin** proteins that enable the specific attachment of the bacterium to its target
- **sex pili**: straighter, thicker and longer than fimbriae; a pilus can extend from one cell to another 'receptive' bacterium and allows the transfer of plasmid DNA.

Bacteria have characteristic shapes (cocci, rods, spirals, etc.) and often occur in characteristic aggregates (e.g. pairs, chains, tetrads, clusters; Fig. 3.3.3). These traits are usually typical for a genus and are diagnostically useful. There are a few bacteria that do not take up the Gram stain and for these special detection methods are used (Fig. 3.3.4):

- *Mycobacterium* spp. have a thick waxy coat that can be detected by the Ziehl–Neelsen stain
- the spirochaetes (*Borrelia*, *Leptospira* and *Treponema* spp.) can be visualized by dark field microscopy
- *Chlamydia*, *Rickettsia* and *Mycoplasma* spp. do not have conventional cell walls and require specialized techniques for their visualization and culture.

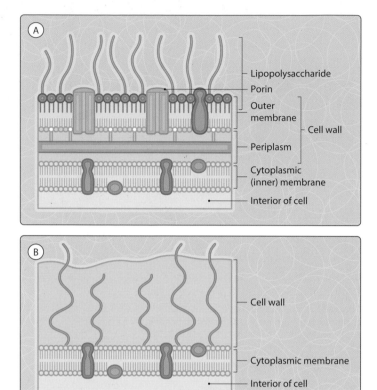

Fig. 3.3.1 Cell wall in Gram-positive (A) and Gram-negative (B) bacteria.

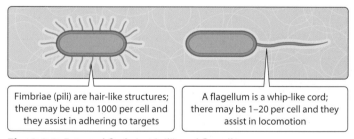

Fimbriae (pili) are hair-like structures; there may be up to 1000 per cell and they assist in adhering to targets

A flagellum is a whip-like cord; there may be 1–20 per cell and they assist in locomotion

Fig. 3.3.2 External fimbriae (pili) and flagellae.

Most bacteria that cause disease grow at human body temperature (37°C). The majority grow in air (**aerobes**) but can grow without it (**facultative anaerobes**); a few can only grow in the absence of oxygen (true **anaerobes**).

Bacteria contain a circular chromosome and extrachromosomal DNA on plasmids. They multiply by **binary fission**, each cell dividing into two 'daughter' cells, and, with division times as short as 20 min, their growth can be explosive from one bacterium to one million within 6 h. Although mutations can occur in chromosomal DNA, their rapid adaptability results from their ability to exchange DNA:

- **transformation**: some bacteria take up DNA from solution outside the cell and incorporate it into their chromosomes

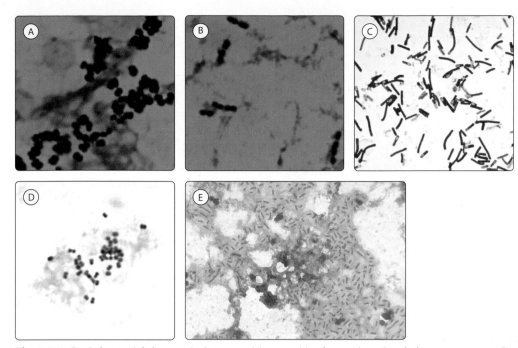

Fig. 3.3.3 Basic bacterial shapes. A. Gram-positive cocci in clumps (e.g. *Staphylococcus aureus, Staphylococcus epidermidis*); B. Gram-positive cocci in chains (e.g. streptococci, enterococci); C. Gram-positive rods (e.g. *Listeria, Bacillus, Corynebacteria, Clostridium* (anaerobic)); D. Gram-negative cocci (e.g. *Neisseria, Moraxella, Veillonella* (anaerobic)); E. Gram-negative rods (e.g. Enterobacteriaceae (*Escherichia. coli, Klebsiella, Salmonella*), *Pseudomonas, Haemophilus, Bacteroides* (anaerobic), *Legionella*).

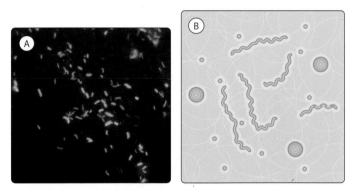

Fig. 3.3.4 Special techniques to visualize bacteria. A. Acid-fast bacteria in Auramine fluorescent stain (e.g. mycobacteria, nocardia); B. non-stainable bacteria in dark-field microscopy (e.g. *Treponema pallidum, Borrellia, Leptospira*).

- **conjugation**: many bacterial cells contain small circular pieces of DNA, called **plasmids**, in addition to their chromosome; plasmids may contain genes for virulence factors and antibiotic resistance, and they can move from one bacterial cell to another
- **transduction**: bacterial cells can be infected by specialized viruses, called **bacteriophages** or **phages**, which move between cells, sometimes carrying genes for virulence factors.

4. Fungi: the basic facts

Questions
- What are mycoses and what types occur?
- In addition to infections, how else can fungi cause disease?

Medically important fungi are eukaryotic organisms and include the **yeasts** (unicellular organisms), **moulds** (filamentous fungi) and **dimorphic fungi** (moulds that transform into yeasts at body temperature). They are widely distributed in the environment and can survive in extreme conditions where nutrients are limited. Most fungi are saprophytes (living off dead organic matter) in soil and water. Certain fungi are also of great commercial value in the production of bread, alcohol and antibiotics.

Yeasts (e.g. *Candida albicans*) are the simplest of the fungi. They are unicellular, spherical in shape and reproduce by budding (Fig. 3.4.1A). In some yeasts, including the medically important genus *Candida*, the buds elongate to form filaments (**pseudohyphae**) (Fig. 3.4.1B).

Moulds are composed of numerous microscopic branching, filamentous **hyphae** (e.g. *Aspergillus fumigatus*; Fig. 3.4.1C,D), known collectively as **mycelia**; these are involved in gaining nutrients and reproduction. The reproductive mycelia produce spores, termed **conidia**, either asexually or by sexual reproduction from opposite mating strains. Spores are disseminated in the atmosphere, enabling fungi to colonize new environments.

Certain pathogenic fungi are **dimorphic** (e.g. *Histoplasma capsulatum*), being a yeast form when invading tissues at 37°C but a mould when living in the environment (room temperature).

Diseases caused by fungi

The study of fungi is called mycology, and the diseases they cause are termed mycoses. Mycoses are classified depending on the degree of tissue involvement and mode of entry into the host:
- superficial: localized to the epidermis, hair and nails but can extend deeper into keratinized tissue
- subcutaneous: confined to the dermis, subcutaneous tissue or adjacent structures
- systemic: deep infections of the internal organs caused by:
  – primary pathogenic fungi, which infect previously healthy persons
  – opportunistic fungi, of marginal pathogenicity but infect the immunocompromised hosts.

Superficial mycoses are the most common mycoses in humans and are acquired from the environment, other infected humans or natural animal hosts. Fungi that invade deeper into keratinized cells are termed dermatophytes. These diseases are often called **tinea** or **ringworm** because of the characteristic red inflammation with central clearing that forms at the site of infection. Dermatophyte infection affects various sites such as the scalp, foot ('athlete's foot') and groin. Although becoming less common, athlete's foot is still the most common fungal infection in the UK. Infections such as pityriasis versicolor (caused by *Malassezia furfur*) are more common in the tropics.

Yeast infections are most commonly caused by *C. albicans* and are confined to the genital tract, mouth and skin folds (**candidiasis** or 'thrush'). This fungus is a commensal of the genital tract and gastrointestinal tract, but it can flourish if ill health, impaired immunity or antibiotic treatment alters the normal bacterial flora.

Subcutaneous mycoses are infections caused by a number of different fungi that arise from injury to the skin. They usually involve the dermis, subcutaneous tissues, muscle and even bone. The fungi commonly live saprophytically on thorn bushes, roses and tree bark, from which wounds can occur. Certain occupational groups (e.g. florists and agricultural workers) are more at risk from infection. Such mycoses are difficult to treat and may require surgical intervention.

Systemic (deep) mycoses are life-threatening invasive infections caused by a variety of fungi. Primary pathogenic fungi infect previously healthy persons and are mainly caused by dimorphic fungi, which are normally found in soil. Infection usually arises from inhaling spores, and the lungs are the main site of infection. However, dissemination to other organs and the central nervous system (CNS) can occur. The incidence is largely confined to endemic areas in North and South America. **Opportunistic fungi** infect vulnerable individuals, who usually have some serious immune or metabolic defect, are taking broad-spectrum antibiotics or immunosuppressive drugs, or have undergone major surgery.

Other fungi-related diseases

Certain fungi may indirectly cause human infections. Constant exposure to fungal spores in the atmosphere can induce respiratory allergies, particularly among certain occupational groups (e.g. farmer's lung). Some mushrooms and toadstools cause poisoning if ingested. Certain moulds produce toxic secondary metabolites (**mycotoxins**) that can contaminate food.

Diagnosis and treatment

The diagnosis and treatment of common mycoses and related diseases is by microscopy and culture of lesions or serology. Antifungal agents are discussed in Chapter 43.

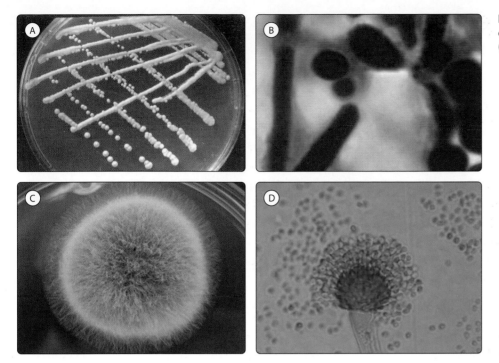

Fig. 3.4.1 Culture plates and microscopy of yeasts (A,B; *Candida* spp.) and moulds (C,D; *Aspergillus* spp., filamentous fungi).

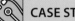 **CASE STUDY: Fungal infection**

A 47-year-old mother had been seeing her GP because of extreme tiredness, bleeding gums and increased bruising. A full blood count showed an abnormal high white blood cell count, low platelets and low haemoglobin. She was referred to the haematology clinic where a bone marrow biopsy was taken and the diagnosis of acute monocytic leukaemia was made. The patient was admitted to hospital the following day and a course of chemotherapy with daunorubicin and cytosine arabinoside (Ara-C) was started. An allograft bone marrow transplantation from one of her teenage children was planned for the near future but unfortunately no remission was achieved despite a second course of chemotherapy. A more immunosuppressive chemotherapy regimen with fludarabine had to be started.

Three weeks after chemotherapy, the patient developed a fever (39°C) with no obvious signs or symptoms of infection. There was no cough although a chest X-ray showed some non-specific shadowing near the mediastinum. Blood test demonstrated profound pancytopenia (neutrophils 0.1×10^9/l, lymphocytes 0.2×10^9/l, platelets 15×10^9/l) and raised C-reactive protein (220 mg/l). The patient was admitted to the haematology ward and a set of blood cultures was taken; she was then started on granulocyte colony-stimulating factor to raise the neutrophil count and empirical broad-spectrum antibiotic therapy (piperacillin with tazobactam and gentamicin) for febrile neutropenia.

The bacterial cultures remained negative after 48 hours of treatment but the fever continued. On day 4 of antibiotic treatment, the patient became increasingly short of breath, with a low oxygen saturation. Clarithromycin was added to cover the possibility of a community-acquired pneumonia, although the pneumococcal urinary antigen test was negative. After a further 24 hours of antibiotic therapy, the patient became increasingly restless, more short of breath and developed a small haemoptysis, which was sent for culture.

The patient had now been neutropenic for more than 21 days and the possibility of an invasive fungal infection was raised. High-resolution computed tomography (HR-CT) of the chest was, therefore, requested. In the immunocompromised, chest radiographs can remain normal or show non-specific signs, whereas the HR-CT is more likely to show subtle changes. The CT indicated two large pulmonary infiltrates close to the mediastinum and a 'halo sign', which is highly suggestive of invasive pulmonary aspergillosis. An intravenous infusion of liposomal amphotericin B was started. Renal function was monitored as this agent can cause nephrotoxicity. The blood-stained sputum grew *Aspergillus fumigatus*, in keeping with invasive pulmonary aspergillosis. Over the following 2 weeks, temperature and inflammatory markers settled and the patient's neutrophil count improved. After a total treatment of 4 weeks with intravenous amphotericin B, the patient was placed on oral voriconazole (an azole active against *Aspergillus*) for a further 2 weeks. A repeat HR-CT showed cavitation of the lesions, which is a sign of resolving infection. The danger is that the fungal infection may reactivate if the patient required further chemotherapy or immunosupression at a later date, which could be fatal.

5. Protozoa: the basic facts

Questions
- How do protozoa move?
- Which protozoa are transmitted by the faecal–oral route?

Protozoa, from the Greek meaning 'first animal', refers to simple, eukaryotic organisms composed of a microscopic single cell. Reproduction is through simple asexual cell division, **binary fission**, in which two daughter cells are formed or **multiple fission**, in which many daughter cells are formed, Certain protozoa have complex life cycles involving both asexual (**schizogony**) and sexual reproduction. Some protozoa form resistant cysts that can survive in the environment.

There are over 65 000 known species of protozoa, of which approximately 10 000 are parasites, deriving nourishment and environmental protection from inhabiting a living animal host. However, the majority of parasites are non-pathogenic, living as harmless commensals within the host. Only a small number of protozoa cause human disease but those that do affect millions of people worldwide, causing considerable suffering, mortality and economic hardship (Table 3.5.1). Protozoal diseases are largely confined to countries with poor economic and social structure. However, trichomoniasis, crytosporidiosis and toxoplasmosis are common in developed countries. Some protozoa of medical importance are described in Chapters 32 and 33.

The pathogenic protozoa are part of the subkingdom Protozoa. Those of medical importance are placed in the phyla Sarcomastigophora, Apicomplexa and Ciliophora. Within these phyla, the protozoa are divided into four major classes based on their locomotive form: the amoebae (Sarcodina), the flagellates (Mastigophora), the sporozoa and the ciliates (Kinetofragminophorea). Examples of common pathogenic protozoa are shown in Fig. 3.5.1.

Amoebae

The amoebae are the simplest of the protozoa and are characterized by a feeding and dividing trophozoite stage that moves by temporary extensions of the cell called **pseudopodia** ('false feet'). In some species, the trophozoite can form a resistant **cyst** stage, which is able to survive in the environment. Those that infect the gut are true parasites, being unable to reproduce except in a living host (e.g. *Entamoeba histolytica*). Others occur naturally in soil and water and are not true parasites. They are termed 'free-living' and infect humans as opportunistic pathogens, for example *Naegleria fowleri* and *Acanthamoeba* sp., the latter causing keratitis in contact lens wearers.

Flagellates

The flagellates have a trophozoite form but also possess flagella for locomotion and food gathering. All pathogenic species are true parasites, being unable to reproduce outside the host. *Trichomonas vaginalis* causes colpitis and *Giardia lamblia* causes gastroenteritis. Pathogenic *Leishmania* spp. and *Trypanosoma* spp. are described in Chapters 32 and 44.

Table 3.5.1 PROTOZOAL INFECTIONS

Organism	Disease and site of infection	Mode of transmission
Amoebae		
Entamoeba histolytica	Amoebiasis; gut and occasionally liver	Faecal–oral route for cysts
Acanthamoeba sp.	Keratitis; eye	Contact lenses, trauma
Naegleria fowleri	Chronic encephalitis in immunocompromised host	Water spread
Flagellates		
Trichomonas vaginalis	Trichomoniasis; vagina and urethra	Sexually transmitted
Giardia lamblia	Giardiasis; gut	Faecal–oral route
Trypanosoma	Trypanosomiasis (Chagas' disease); fever, lymphadenopathy, hepatosplenopathy, heart disease	Insect bite (tsetse fly)
Leishmania spp.	Leishmaniasis; skin, mucocutaneous surfaces, viscera (liver, spleen), bone marrow	Insect bite (sandfly)
Ciliates		
Balantidium coli	Balantidiosis; gut	Soil
Apicomplexa		
Plasmodium spp.	Malaria; erythrocytes, liver	Insect bite (female *Anopheles* mosquito)
Cryptosporidium parvum	Cryptosporidiosis; gut	Faecal–oral route
Toxoplasma gondii	Toxoplasmosis; systemic flu like illness in immunocompetent; heart and CNS in immunosuppressed; CNS and eye in congenital infection	Cat faeces, undercooked meat, transplacental, organ transplant

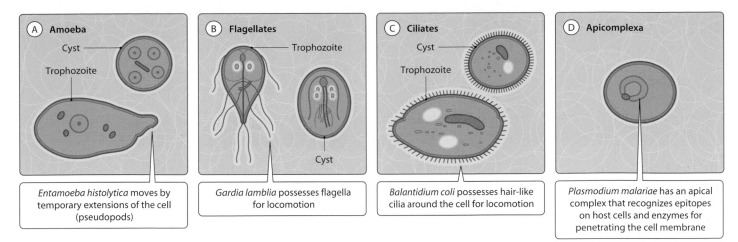

Fig. 3.5.1 Examples of human pathogenic protozoa. A. Amoebae (e.g. *Entamoeba histolytica*); B. flagellates (e.g. *Giardia lamblia*); C. ciliates (e.g. *Balantidium coli*); D. apicomplexa (e.g. *Plasmodium malariae*).

Ciliates

The ciliates possess rows of hair-like cilia around the outside of the body for motility and also to direct food into a primitive mouth, termed a cytostome. All ciliates possess two nuclei: a large polyploid micronucleus and a small micronucleus active only during sexual reproduction. Some species form cysts (e.g. *Balantidium coli*, which causes colitis).

Apicomplexa

Apicomplexa is a unique group lacking any visible means of locomotion. They are all parasitic and most are intracellular, having a life cycle involving both sexual and asexual reproduction. The common feature of all members is the presence of an **apical complex** (visible only by electron microscopy) at the anterior pole in one or more stages of the life cycle. The exact components of the apical complex vary among members. It is thought that it enables cell penetration. This group comprises *Plasmodium* spp. (Ch. 33), *Toxoplasma gondii* (Chs 31 and 35) and *Cryptosporidium parvum* (Ch 32).

Diagnosis

The relatively large size of the protozoa enables most human pathogens to be easily identified by microscopic examination of clinical material. Those of the gut are observed in freshly taken faecal samples. Blood and tissue protozoa are visualized after staining. Detection of elevated antibodies to the infecting organism may be diagnostic in some instances (e.g. toxoplasmosis). Culture methods are not routinely used as they are technically demanding and time consuming: an exception is the diagnosis of trichomoniasis. Treatment is described in Chapter 44.

6. Helminths: the basic facts

Questions
- Which are the three major classes of pathogenic helminth?
- Which classes of helminth possess a mouth and digestive system?

Helminths (from the Greek *helminthos*, meaning worm) refers to all parasitic worms of humans. They are complex, multicellular organisms, ranging in size from the microscopic filarial parasites to the giant tapeworms, several metres in length. Sexual reproduction occurs in all, usually by mating between male and female larvae. However, some helminths are hermaphroditic, possessing both male and female reproductive organs and can reproduce by self-fertilization, termed parthenogenesis.

Human helminth diseases occur worldwide but are most prevalent in countries with poor socioeconomic development. They seldom cause acute disease but produce chronic infections that can have a severely debilitating effect on the host (Ch. 34).

Parasitic helminths comprise the **nematodes** (roundworms, filaria), **cestodes** (tapeworms) and **trematodes** (flukes) (Fig. 3.6.1).

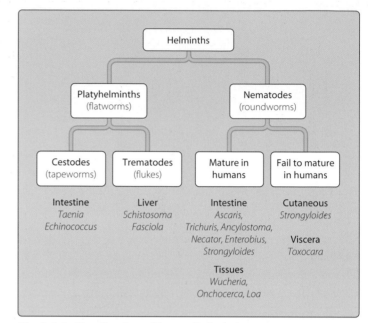

Fig. 3.6.1 Classification of human helminths.

Nematodes

The nematodes are typically worm-like in appearance (Fig. 3.6.2). The intestinal pathogenic nematodes may be divided into two groups.

Those that develop in soil, the larvae being the infectious stage.   The larvae are shed in the faeces and mature in the soil. They infect humans by burrowing into the skin (usually through the soles of the feet) and enter the bloodstream to be carried to the heart and lungs. They then force their way into the alveolus and trachea, and, on reaching the epiglottis, are swallowed. The life cycle then continues in the small intestine.

Those that survive in soil, the eggs being infective.   The eggs are the infectious form in which the larvae develop. When ingested, the larvae hatch in the small intestine, penetrate the mucosa and are carried through the bloodstream to the heart and lungs. The rest of the life cycle is as described above.

In other nematodes the eggs hatch in the intestine, where the worms develop and produce eggs, which are shed in the faeces. The larvae can sometimes migrate through the body to infect other organs.

Filaria

The filaria are microscopic nematodes, transmitted by biting insect vectors in which part of the nematode's life cycle is completed. On infecting humans, the larvae mate and the females produce **microfilariae**, which develop in the blood, lymphatic system, skin and eye. This can result in gross swelling of infected tissues, most notably in the groin and legs.

Cestodes (tapeworms)

The tapeworms are flat, ribbon-like worms that can grow up to 10 m in length (Fig. 3.6.2B). They produce eggs, which are excreted into the environment and can infect a variety of hosts in which the life cycle continues. Humans become infected from consuming contaminated meat. They are characterized by:

- lack of a mouth, digestive tract and vascular system
- a scolex (head) that attaches to the intestinal wall by suckers
- a tegument (body) of the scolex through which nutrients are absorbed
- proglottids (segments) forming the tegument, each containing male and female reproductive organs and producing infective eggs
- eggs of *Taenia solium*, which hatch in the gut releasing motile larvae; these migrate through the gut wall and blood vessels to encyst in muscle, forming cysticerci (fluid-filled cysts each containing a scolex).

Trematodes (flukes)

The trematodes are flat, leaf-like organisms (Fig. 3.6.2C). They have complicated life cycles, alternating between a sexual reproductive cycle in the final host (humans) and an asexual

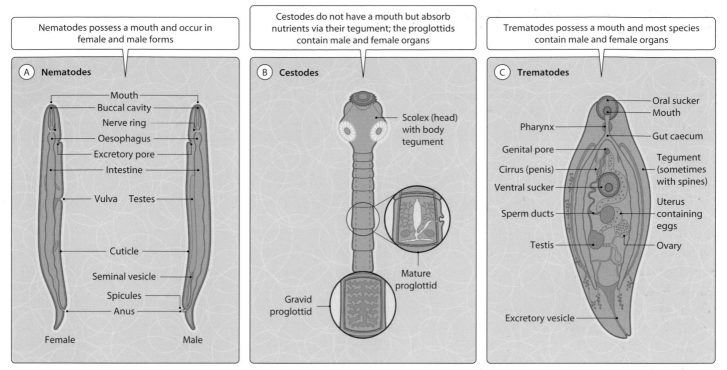

Fig. 3.6.2 Principal features of nematodes (A), cestodes (B) and trematodes (C).

multiplicative cycle in a snail host. They cause infection of the liver, bladder and rectum. Their major features are:

- a mouth and digestive tract but no anus
- hermaphroditic, except for the schistosomes, which have a boat-shaped male and a cylindrical female form
- part of their life cycle is completed in an aquatic snail host.

Diagnosis and treatment

Intestinal helminths are identified by microscopic examination of faeces. Filaria are detected in blood and tissue samples after staining. As with the protozoa, helminth infections are difficult to treat because of the lack of effective agents. Those that are available are toxic and unable to destroy all the various forms (Ch. 44).

CASE STUDY: Helminth infection

A 20-year-old man returned from a 3 month trip through South America and complained of an itchy creeping eruption on his left foot. The erythema had a serpinguous shape (see Fig. 3.32.2). Steroid ointment had improved the pruritus; however, the eruption was still coming and going. In Brazil, he had already received mebendazole, which did not cure it.

The diagnosis is cutaneous larva migrans, which is most commonly caused by the canine hookworm *Ancylostoma braziliensis*.

Dogs or cats excrete eggs into sand on the beach, where larvae hatch and penetrate the skin of humans on contact. The larva remains in the subcutaneous tissues and little further development occurs. Mebendazole does not achieve larvicidal concentrations in the tissues, whereas ivermectin and thiabendazole do. After a single dose of ivermectin, the eruption subsided within a week.

7. Viroids, prions and virinos

Questions
- What are the different properties of viroids, prions and virinos?
- What are the features of the important spongiform/degenerative encephalopathies?

The viroids, prions and virinos are infectious agents that are simpler than viruses.

Viroids

Viroids cause, predominantly, plant diseases such as potato spindle-tuber disease. They consist of circular, single-stranded RNA, usually 250 to 370 nucleotides long. In plants, they are found mainly in the nucleolus, but little else is known of the pathogenic mechanisms that they employ. Human disease caused by viroids is not yet recognized.

Prions

Prions are putative infectious agents, so-called because they are proteinaceous infectious particles (the originator changed it from proin). Although there is not universal agreement that they exist in vivo, the evidence for them is now considerable. The best studied is the prion that causes a degenerative disorder of the CNS of sheep, scrapie. This agent appears to be a 33–35 kDa hydrophobic protein that has been termed PrP (for prion protein). The gene that encodes for this protein exists in normal sheep, but the product in diseased animals has a mutant peptide sequence and an abnormal isoform with β-pleated sheets replacing α-helical domains; the normal cellular protein is termed PrPc, the abnormal PrPsc. The abnormal protein further differs from the normal cellular protein by being insoluble in detergents, highly resistant to proteases and having a tendency to aggregate. Prion proteins have been shown to be infectious and to have a high but not absolute degree of species specificity.

Virinos

An alternative hypothesis for the infectious agent of scrapie has been the virino. This putative agent has a tiny, as yet undetectable, scrapie-specific nucleic acid coated in PrP. There is currently no evidence for the existence of this agent, but it offers a plausible explanation for the strain variation that is known to occur in scrapie.

Transmissible spongiform/degenerative encephalopathies

Scrapie is a transmissible spongiform/degenerative encephalopathy (TSE/TDE) of sheep, and many other ungulates suffer this disorder. The well-publicized cow equivalent is bovine spongiform encephalopathy (BSE). It is now recognized that TDEs also occur in humans. The features of a TDE are:

- the presence of 'holes' in the neuronal matrix (spongiform degeneration) caused by amyloid
- the presence of aggregates of prion proteins into amyloid fibrils (Fig. 3.7.1)
- a long incubation period (several months to many years)
- rapidly progressive
- clinical presentation with cognitive impairment, ataxia, myoclonus and extrapyramidal signs.

The well-characterized human prion diseases are Creutzfeldt–Jakob disease (CJD), variant Creutzfeldt–Jakob disease (vCJD), kuru, Gerstmann–Straüsller–Scheinker (GSS) syndrome and fatal familial insomnia (FFI). GSS and FFI are familial and very rare. Kuru was associated with the cannibalism of human brains in Papua New Guinea and is of historical interest. The tentative diagnosis of human TDE is made from the clinical features, which occur usually in patients between 40 and 70 years of age; vCJD disease, however, involves younger patients and has been strongly associated with the ingestion of meat from cows infected with BSE. Confirmation of the diagnosis currently depends on the neuropathological features found at postmortem, although newer methods based on detection of the abnormal PrP by labelled-specific antibody are becoming more widely available and constitute the definitive test. Currently there is no treatment, so prevention forms the bedrock of control. Brain

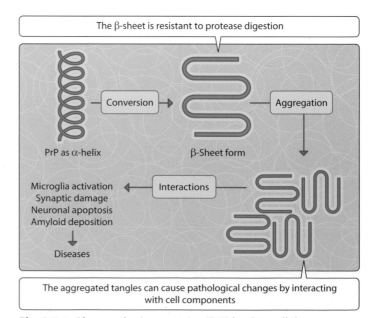

The β-sheet is resistant to protease digestion

PrP as α-helix → Conversion → β-Sheet form → Aggregation

Microglia activation ← Interactions
Synaptic damage
Neuronal apoptosis
Amyloid deposition
↓
Diseases

The aggregated tangles can cause pathological changes by interacting with cell components

Fig. 3.7.1 Abnormal prion proteins (PrP) lead to cell damage, disease and death.

and spinal cord appear to be the predominant reservoir of infection, and transmission has been shown to occur with infected corneal and dura mater grafts, growth hormone and gonadotrophin injections and the use of contaminated neurosurgical instruments. There is also a genetic component to disease susceptibility, with 10% of CJD cases being familial and a higher prevalence of sporadic CJD in, for example, Israeli Jews of Libyan origin. The gene for the human prion protein is located on chromosome 20, and homozygosity at codon 129 (methionine or valine) confers susceptibility to CJD, although this mutation is not directly linked to disease causation. Such markers may be useful in the future for diagnostic and screening purposes.

 CASE STUDY: Prion disease

A 54-year-old woman had suffered poor vision in both eyes for many years. A thorough ophthalmology review concluded that she suffered from a rare autosomal dominant degenerative disorder of her corneal endothelium called Fuchs' endothelial dystrophy. After 1 year of unsuccessful medical treatment she opted for a corneal transplant. She was referred to a specialist corneal transplant unit.

The consultant ophthalmologist asked for her consent to use a cadaveric corneal transplant. As part of the consent procedure, she was informed that she would not be able to donate blood or organs after receiving the corneal graft. The lady was quite upset as she has been a blood donor for many years and asked why this would be the case. The doctor explained that although corneal donors are extensively tested for blood-borne viruses (HIV, hepatitis B and C) and other infectious diseases such as syphilis, there might be a residual risk of transmitting a form of transmissible spongiform encephalopathy (such as variant Creuzfeldt–Jakob disease (CJD)), which is caused by infectious proteinaceous entities called prions. Such diseases can lead to dementia and death. The doctor reassured the patient that only very few cases have been described in the world and that the acquisition of such an infection would be extremely rare. In suspected cases of CJD, a cerebrospinal sample can be tested for an abnormal protein (14-3-3 protein), but ultimately only a brain or possibly tonsil biopsy would confirm such diagnosis.

8. Epidemiology of infectious diseases

Questions
■ Contrast the main routes of transmission of infectious disease
■ What are the differences between endemic and epidemic outbreaks?

Epidemiology is 'the study of the occurrence, distribution and control of disease in populations'. The risk of infection depends upon more than simply an individual's susceptibility; it is also affected by the level of disease within the population, the degree of population mixing and 'herd immunity', as well as specific features such as the communicable period, route and ease (infectiousness) of transmission.

Route of transmission
For an infectious agent to persist within a population there must be a *cycle* of transmission from a contaminated source, through a portal of entry, into a susceptible host and on again (Fig. 3.8.1).
Direct transmission. This is the most common and important route. It involves all forms of physical contact between humans, including sexual transmission, faecal–oral spread and direct respiratory spread via large droplets.
Vector-borne transmission. Infection is mediated by arthropods or insects; it is mechanical if the vector is simply a source of contamination, but biological if the vector is necessary for the multiplication or maturation of the infectious agent.
Vehicle-borne transmission. This describes spread from all contaminated inanimate objects. Vehicles include clothing, food, water, surgical instruments and also biological substances such as blood and tissues.
Air-borne transmission.   Aerosols suspended in the air for long periods can be a source of infection.
Animal-borne infections.   A **zoonosis** is any infection spread from a vertebrate animal to a human.

Disease in the population
Prevalence is 'the number of cases of infection per unit of population at a single point in time'.

Incidence refers to 'the number of new cases of infection per unit of population over a specified period of time'. For **acute** infections, lasting only a few days or possibly weeks, the incidence may be very high but the prevalence relatively low. However, for **chronic** infections, lasting months or years, the prevalence may be relatively high even though the incidence is low. Infections like urinary tract infections occur at roughly

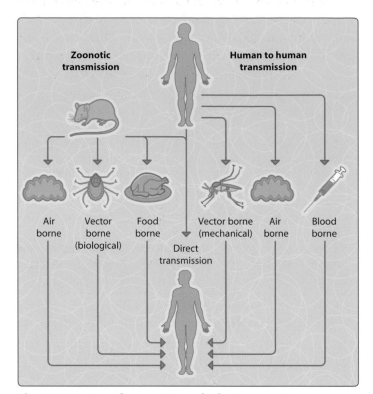

Fig. 3.8.1 Routes of transmission of infectious agents.

steady levels throughout the year; other infections may vary, for example the rise in respiratory tract infections during the winter. The **periodicity** of some infections is measured over a much longer scale, for example the roughly 4 year cycle in *Mycoplasma* pneumonias.

Infections that have a stable incidence within the population are described as **endemic** (or **hyperendemic** if the incidence is extremely high). Cases are frequently unconnected and are then referred to as **sporadic**. A number of terms are used to describe situations in which the *number of infections is greater than that which might be anticipated from previous experience.*
Outbreak. A cluster of cases in a single household or over a small area is described as an outbreak. It may relate to exposure to a local source, and suitable detective work and control procedures may prevent further transmission.
Epidemic. An increase in cases over a larger region, perhaps an entire country, is described as an epidemic. This is less likely to be caused by a single source, and more extensive measures will be required to control the spread.
Pandemic. If the increase occurs over a larger area still, at least several countries, it is described as a pandemic.
The burden of infectious diseases varies enormously throughout the world, dependent upon factors such as environmental

conditions, wealth and nutritional status, local human behaviour and the efficiency of healthcare. Examples of the variation in prevalence of some of the common infectious diseases globally is shown in Fig. 3.8.2. Health service managers clearly need this information to plan for the future; however, it is vital that *every clinician* be aware of local and regional patterns of disease in order to achieve effective diagnosis, treatment and control of infection within their own practice area. For serious communicable diseases in the UK, **surveillance** is achieved through a *legal requirement* for medical practitioners to inform the local 'consultant in communicable disease control' (or the 'consultant in public health medicine' in Scotland) of *all* cases of **notifiable disease** (Appendix, Table A.3). For less-serious infections, individual general practices or hospital units may volunteer to report their cases of infection through government or professional association programmes.

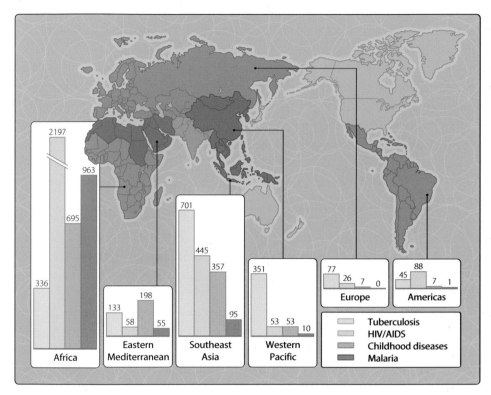

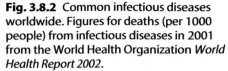

Fig. 3.8.2 Common infectious diseases worldwide. Figures for deaths (per 1000 people) from infectious diseases in 2001 from the World Health Organization *World Health Report 2002.*

9. Pathogenesis of infectious disease

Questions
- What are the basic determinants of pathogenicity?
- What are Koch's postulates?
- Compare the mechanisms whereby microorganisms evade host defences.

Contamination of the body occurs when a microorganism becomes in contact with a host and this becomes **colonization** when the organism multiplies. Only a minority of microorganisms are in contact with humans, and most of these are commensal flora within their own ecological niche. However, viruses and other pathogenic microorganisms characteristically cause disease; they may have highly specific adhesins and toxins, the genes for which may be grouped together under the control of a single promoter in **pathogenicity islands**. The net result of the meeting between a human and any microorganism depends on the balance between **host immunity** and the **virulence** of the infectious agent. **Commensalism** occurs when there is a neutral balance between the two parties, **symbiosis** when both benefit and **parasitism** when the relationship is uneven. However, interaction with microorganisms occurs continually, the relationship can change and disease is common. So, how do we know if the two are linked? **Koch's postulates** are an important set of criteria that can be used to judge whether a microorganism is the cause of a disease. They can be summarized (with a slight change in emphasis from the original treatise of Koch) as:

1. The organism occurs in every case of the disease and under circumstances which account for the pathological changes and clinical course of the disease
2. The organism occurs in other diseases as a fortuitous and non-pathogenic finding
3. After being isolated from the body and grown in pure culture, the organism can repeatedly produce exactly the same disease when inoculated into new, susceptible hosts
4. The organism can then be isolated from the new hosts.

These postulates are still relevant today, although it is difficult to apply them to poorly demarcated clinical syndromes such as diseases where the pathogen that initiated a disease process is no longer present, as occurs in some autoimmune diseases; malignancies; multifactorial diseases; serious diseases without an animal model; infections in the immunocompromised; and uncultivatable microorganisms. An understanding of molecular mechanisms has also shown that the same bacterium can be pathogenic and non-pathogenic depending on differential gene expression.

In order to cause an infection, a microorganism has to make contact with the host (Fig. 3.9.1), multiply within it and then be transmitted to another host/area.

Contact and adhesion

Infectious agents must gain entry to the host and stick to target tissues. Portals of entry include the gastrointestinal tract, respiratory mucosa, genital mucosa and direct inoculation through the skin.

Many agents have **adhesins** on their surface or on **fimbriae** that project from the cell. Parasites may even physically hold on to their host (Table 3.9.1). Adhesion will protect microorganisms from the flushing of mucosal surfaces. Gastrointestinal pathogens have some resistance to gastric acid and bile, while agents of skin infections are resistant to drying.

Evasion of host defences/production of virulence factors

Microorganisms that successfully invade host tissues increase their numbers by producing a range of factors that enable them to survive the onslaught of innate and specific immunity and which are responsible for the development of clinical disease.

Toxins (Table 3.9.2) are substances that can damage a host's cells and which may be active away from the site of production. An **exotoxin** is secreted, while an **endotoxin** is a constitutive part of the pathogen, in particular the **lipopolysaccharide** (LPS) of the Gram-negative bacterial cell wall. Toxins may be subdivided further, for example according to their cellular target, their mode of action or their biological effect. Some toxins, such as toxic shock syndrome toxin 1, have an additional effect of acting as superantigens, causing polyclonal activation and cytokine release to impair an effective immune response. If developing T cells are exposed, deletion of that clone results.

Other virulence factors may be produced locally without causing cellular damage. For example, some *Staphylococcus aureus* strains may produce a **coagulase** that coagulates fibrinogen and increases the likelihood of abscess formation, while others may produce a **hyaluronidase**, which breaks down intercellular junctions, leading to cellulitis. Different species of bacteria produce different kinases, lecithinases and proteases, which partly explains the range in virulence and clinical presentation of the various agents.

Other factors include **siderophores**, which steal essential iron from host carrier proteins; secreted surface **capsules**, which reduce phagocytic efficiency; factors preventing phagosome–lysozome fusion; and substances that allow the pathogen to escape from the phagosome into the host cytoplasm.

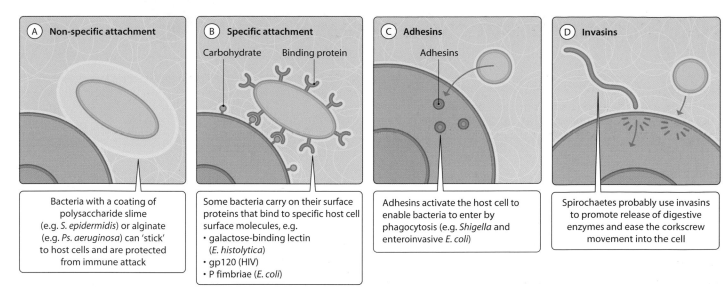

Fig. 3.9.1 Methods of attachment used by microbes.

Table 3.9.1 EXAMPLES OF ADHESION OF INFECTIOUS AGENTS

Agent	Mechanism
Non-specific methods	
Giardia lamblia	Mechanical 'gripping disc'
Staphylococcus epidermidis	Polysaccharide slime
Pseudomonas aeroginosa	Alginate production
Specific methods (adhesins)	
Entamoeba histolytica	Galactose-binding lectin
Escherichia coli	P fimbriae (binding to uroepithelial cells, P blood group antigen)
Yersinia enterocolitica	Ail protein (binding to epithelial integrin)
Human immunodeficiency virus	gp120 (binding to CD4 antigen)

Transmission

To complete the cycle of infection, infectious agents will need to be excreted, the route dictating the mechanism of spread:

- faecal–oral spread involves excretion within stool samples and may be aided by the production of copious volumes of hygiene-challenging diarrhoea
- spread via the respiratory tract as respiratory tract secretions, often aerosolized by sneezing and coughing
- spread in vaginal/cervical or urethral discharges, which will transmit infection by sexual contact.

Zoonotic infections are transmitted in diverse ways when the human is a normal part of the infectious cycle. They include the obvious methods of discharge, such as excretion of the agent in faeces and urine, but also via **parasitaemia**, which helps to ensure uptake by blood-sucking insects (e.g. anopholene mosquitos and malaria), and the budding of rabies virus from the apical surfaces of salivary gland epithelia, which accounts for spread via the bite of a rabid animal.

Table 3.9.2 EXAMPLES OF BACTERIAL TOXINS

Name	Source	Receptor	Biological effect
Cholera toxin	*Vibrio cholerae*	GM1 ganglioside	Activation of adenylyl cyclase; secretory diarrhoea
Diphtheria toxin	*Corynebacterium diphtheriae*	Epidemal growth factor-like precursor	Inhibition of protein synthesis, cell death
Oedema factor	*Corynebacterium anthracis*	Unknown glycoprotein	Increase in target cell cAMP, haemolysis
Shiga toxin	*Shigella dysenteriae*	Globotriaosyl ceramide	Reduced protein synthesis, cell death
Tetanus toxin	*Clostridium tetani*	Ganglioside	Reduced release of neurotransmitters, spastic paralysis
Toxic shock syndrome toxin I	*Staphylococcus aureus*	T-cell receptor	Acts as a superantigen causing uncoordinated immune stimulation

10. Pathology of infectious disease

Questions
■ By what mechanisms do microorganisms damage tissues?
■ How does the host respond pathologically to infection?

Symptoms of infection arise from direct damage to tissues, 'poisoning of cells', immune-mediated damage (immunopathology) or a combination of these. Subclinical infection may occur, however, without any such damage. Disease severity depends on both host factors and virulence determinants of the microorganism. Host determinants of disease severity include age, nutritional status, genetic constitution, immune status, local environment (e.g. gastric pH), presence of normal flora and presence of physical barriers (such as intact skin). Factors that affect the virulence of a pathogen include the infectious titre, the route of entry and genetic expression (e.g. of virulence factors). Both host and microbial factors can be altered by environmental changes such as ambient temperature and use of antibiotics. Even in an outbreak arising from a single pathogen, there is often a spectrum of clinical presentation.

Damage to tissues

Most viruses cause damage to the cells they infect. Viruses abort host replicative mechanisms and may thus cause death of the cell or, when mature, they may lyse the cell as they erupt. If a large fraction of the cells is infected, then there is extensive tissue damage. Programmed cell death (**apoptosis**) is also now recognized as a common mechanism that many viruses, such as HIV and influenza A, use to cause cell damage.

Macroscopically, extensive tissue necrosis is, however, rare, and patchy necrosis with oedema owing to membrane damage is all that is seen. Viral infection is also characterized by changes in the cytoskeleton and organelles. There may be shrinkage of the nucleus (**pyknosis**) and aggregations of newly formed virus may be seen as **inclusion bodies**. Some viruses, such as paramyxoviruses, also cause cell-to-cell fusion to yield multinucleate cells.

Viruses such as hepatitis B virus, herpesviruses (particularly Epstein–Barr virus) and papillomaviruses are known to be oncogenic. The precise mechanisms of cancer causation are not fully elucidated but genes that provide oncogenic potential have been identified; for example, the product of the *X* gene of hepatitis B virus has been shown to inhibit DNA repair mechanisms and, therefore, allow the accumulation of mutations.

Bacteria may exist intracellularly within phagocytic cells. These cells may then be destroyed. Parenchymal cells are,

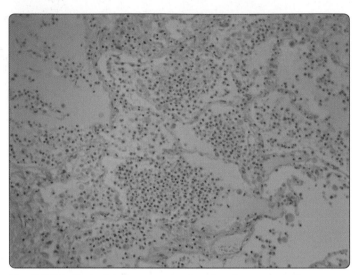

Fig. 3.10.1 Bacterial pneumonia, showing the acute inflammatory response.

however, more commonly damaged by extracellular products such as toxins, enzymes and pH change. *Helicobacter pylori*, for example, produces urease, which causes hydrogen ion changes, and mucinase, which degrades the protective mucous layer of the stomach cavity; both of these mechanisms are thought to contribute to the cell damage that results in gastritis and peptic ulceration.

Cell toxicity

Viruses can be broadly considered as cell poisons. Bacteria exert most of their direct cell and tissue damage through the production of toxins. The end result tends to be loss of function, which might be manifest as oedema and necrosis of tissue but may not have macroscopic effects. Some fungi can also produce toxins, a well-characterized example being aflatoxin produced by *Aspergillus flavus*, which contaminates monkey nuts.

Inflammation and immunopathology

There are four types of immunopathological reaction: type 1 is IgE mediated, type 2 is complement-mediated, type 3 is immune-complex mediated and type 4 is a delayed cytotoxic reaction caused by T cells. Acute inflammation with an influx of neutrophils and other inflammatory cells can produce obvious changes in tissues (Fig. 3.10.1). If this is extensive, then long-term fibrotic changes may result. Immunopathology can result from these different types of immune reaction to infection (Fig. 3.10.2). The cell-mediated immune response to *Mycobacterium tuberculosis* results in characteristic pathology, with granulomata exhibiting central caseous (cheesy) necrosis (Fig. 3.10.3).

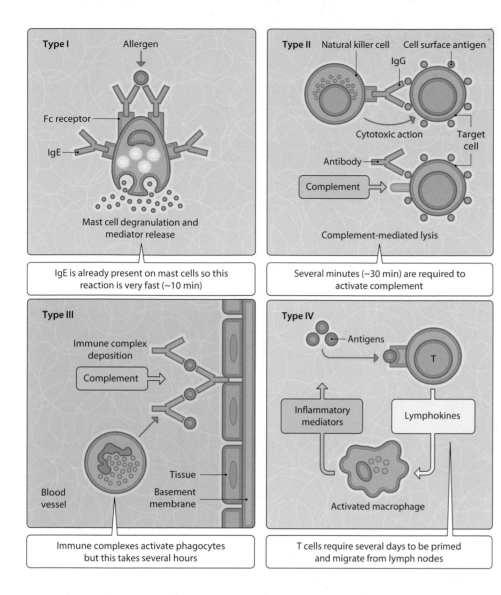

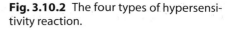

Fig. 3.10.2 The four types of hypersensitivity reaction.

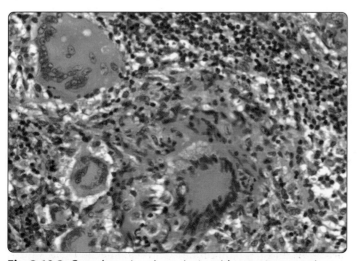

Fig. 3.10.3 Granuloma in tuberculosis, with caseous necrosis.

The production of autoantibodies (e.g. to DNA or erythrocytes) is not uncommon, but overt **autoimmune** disease occurs as a result of few infections: examples include rheumatic fever as a result of infection with group A streptococci, thyroiditis resulting from enterovirus infection and arthritis as a reaction to chlamydial or salmonella infection. Simplistically, these arise because of molecular mimicry between host components and foreign antigens, with an immune response initially directed against an antigen on the microbe then recognizing a similar structure of a host component as foreign.

11. Innate host defences to infectious disease

Questions
- What are the innate (non-specific) defences?
- What is the role of phagocytes in infection?
- Describe the sources and roles of cytokines.

The skin and mucous membranes are physical barriers that form the first defence against infection (Fig. 3.11.1). They have high cell turnover, with superficial cells, which may have become colonized by pathogens, constantly being shed. Most sites are further protected by secretions of **mucus**, which trap microorganisms and prevent them sticking directly to epithelial cells, and substances such as lysozyme (a powerful degradative enzyme) and lactoferrin (an iron-binding protein that makes the essential acquisition of iron by bacteria difficult). Environments may be made more hostile still by an acid pH, such as in the stomach, vagina or urine, or by alkaline pH, such as in the duodenum. It is also difficult for microorganisms to rest on epithelial surfaces because of the peristalsis of gut contents, periodic flushing of the urethra with urine and the muco-ciliary escalator of the respiratory tract. The normal bacterial flora at many of these sites can also be protective against incoming pathogens because of several factors:

- scavenging of all available nutrients
- maintenance of hostile conditions, e.g. *Lactobacillus* spp. metabolism contributes to the acid pH of the vagina
- natural production of 'antibiotics' (**bacteriocins**)
- direct cell-to-cell contact inhibition
- ensuring 'fitness' of specific immunity by subclinical stimulation at mucosal sites.

Within tissues, **phagocytic cells** ingest microorganisms into **phagosomes**, which then merge with intracytoplasmic granules (**lysosomes**) containing toxic reagents to form **phagolysosomes**, where the microorganisms will be killed by oxygen-dependent and oxygen-independent mechanisms (Fig. 3.11.2):

- oxygen independent: lysozyme, acid hydrolases, cationic proteins, lactoferrin, neutral proteases
- oxygen dependent: hydrogen peroxide, singlet oxygen, hydroxyl radical, hypothalite, nitric oxide.

These **antigen-presenting cells** then channel the breakdown products from the phagocytosed microorganisms onto their surface, where they are made available for stimulation of passing cells from the specific immune system. **Natural killer** cells are cytotoxic cells related to T lymphocytes, but as they act non-specifically and without memory they are included here.

A number of **acute-phase proteins** are produced in response to infection, including the **complement system**. This series of proteins is sequentially activated, with some of the later products of the cascade amplifying the activation of earlier components through positive feedback. The process may be initiated directly by contact with microorganisms (**alternative** and **mannan-binding lectin** pathways) or through recognition of antibody–antigen complexes (**classic** pathway). The later stages of the cascade and the net results are the same regardless of the mechanism of activation. Complement factors are deposited onto the microbe's surface or liberated into the site of infection with the following effects:

- **inflammation**: some products are chemotactic factors that attract more cells of the immune system to the area
- **opsonization**: some factors, when deposited on the surface of microorganisms, improve phagocytic efficiency
- **lysis**: the terminal components of the complement system form a ring-like structure on the surface of infectious agents, which punches a hole in the membrane, leading to death of the pathogen.

Although the above elements provide innate or non-specific immunity, in practice they act in conjunction with parts of the

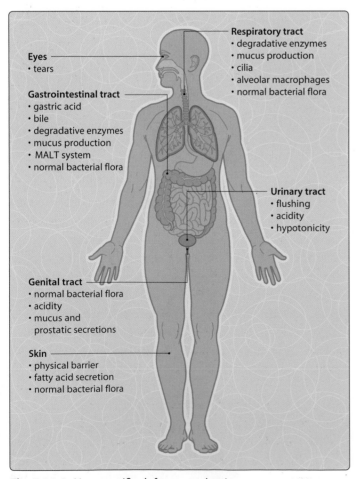

Eyes
- tears

Gastrointestinal tract
- gastric acid
- bile
- degradative enzymes
- mucus production
- MALT system
- normal bacterial flora

Genital tract
- normal bacterial flora
- acidity
- mucus and prostatic secretions

Skin
- physical barrier
- fatty acid secretion
- normal bacterial flora

Respiratory tract
- degradative enzymes
- mucus production
- cilia
- alveolar macrophages
- normal bacterial flora

Urinary tract
- flushing
- acidity
- hypotonicity

Fig. 3.11.1 Non-specific defence mechanisms.

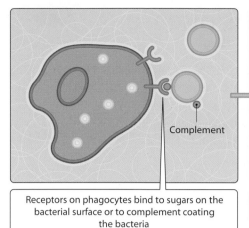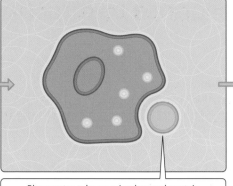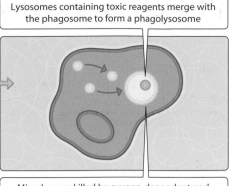

Lysosomes containing toxic reagents merge with the phagosome to form a phagolysosome

Complement

Receptors on phagocytes bind to sugars on the bacterial surface or to complement coating the bacteria

Phagocytes take up microbes and contain them in phagosomes

Microbes are killed by oxygen-dependent and oxygen-independent mechanisms

Fig. 3.11.2 Phagocytosis and intracellular killing.

Table 3.11.1 SOURCES AND EFFECTS OF SOME CYTOKINES

Cytokine	Source	Target	Action
IL-1	Macrophages	Lymphocytes, phagocytes	General activation
		Hepatocytes	Synthesis of acute phase proteins
IL-6	Macrophages, CD4 T cells	B cells	
		Hepatocytes	Synthesis of acute phase proteins (liver)
IFN-α	Monocytes	T cells	General activation
		Infected cells	Increased HLA class I expression, inhibition of viral replication
Tumour necrosis factor	T cells, monocytes	Lymphocytes, phagocytes	General activation
		Hepatocytes	Synthesis of acute phase proteins (liver)
IL-2	CD4 cells	T cells	Proliferation, maturation
		Natural killer cells	Activation
IFN-γ	T cells	Macrophages	Activation
		Most cells	Increased HLA class I and II expression
Granulocyte–macrophage colony-stimulating factor	T cells, macrophages, endothelial cells	Granulocytes, macrophages	Increased growth, differentiation of precursors
IL-10	Lymphocytes, macrophages	T cells, macrophages	Inhibited cytokine production
		Antigen-presenting cells	Decreased HLA class II expression

IL, interleukin; IFN, interferon.

adaptive immune system. For example, antigen presentation by phagocytes is essential for T helper cell stimulation; in turn, antibody can act as an opsonin, and cytokine production by activated T helper cells turns on oxygen-dependent killing, both of which improve the efficiency of phagocytosis.

Cytokines (Table 3.11.1) are soluble mediators that produce complex overlapping signals between host cells; they are secreted by monocytes, macrophages and lymphocytes and other cells. Those responsible for communication between cells of the immune system are called interleukins (IL). Cytokines such as IL-1, IL-6 and interferon-α mainly promote non-specific immunity, while IL-2 mainly affects cells of the specific immune system. Tumour necrosis factor and interferon-γ tend to increase inflammation, while granulocyte–monocyte colony-stimulating factor targets precursor cells within the bone marrow. Most cytokines have a stimulatory effect, but IL-10 tends to suppress immune function. There are over 200 cytokines now recognized.

12. Adaptive host response to infectious disease

Questions
- How does a host respond to defend itself from infection?
- Describe the role of different T cells during infection
- What is the function of the Fc fragment of IgG?

In contrast to innate immunity, **acquired, adaptive** or **specific immunity** is both highly specific in its recognition of foreign material and also becomes more efficient with repeated exposure to the same stimulus. The pivotal cell is the **lymphocyte**, which is able to respond to a *single* foreign **antigen**. This clearly requires a massive number of cells if an individual is to be able to react to the huge range of microorganisms that may be encountered in a lifetime. This diversity is generated by having multiple, variable germline genes coding for antigen receptors that recombine in a random manner within each precursor lymphocyte; these cells then mature in early life, by a process of positive and negative selection, to give a mixed population of competent cells that can be activated but which will not react against 'self'. Upon exposure to the appropriate antigen, these cells proliferate and differentiate either into short-acting 'effector' cells or into long-lasting memory cells, which will allow a more rapid and greater response on subsequent exposure to the *same* antigen (Fig. 3.12.1).

Lymphocytes may usefully be divided up into B lymphocytes (humoral immunity) and T lymphocytes (cell-mediated immunity) according to the molecules that they express on their surface, such as the cluster differentiation (CD) markers, and by their pattern of cytokine production. The T helper (Th) cells are subgroups of lymphocytes that are involved in activating and directing other immune cells (e.g. determining B cell antibody class switching, activation and growth of cytotoxic T cells). Mature Th cells express the surface protein CD4 and are known as CD4 T cells (Fig. 3.12.2).

B lymphocytes

Each B lymphocyte has **antibodies** or **immunoglobulins**, specific for just one antigen, arranged facing outwards as receptors on its surface; if exposed to that antigen, the B cell proliferates and then differentiates (Fig. 3.12.1). Its effectors are called **plasma cells**, and each one can only produce antibody of *single* antigen specificity, although the **isotype** may vary as the immune response matures. The basic structure of an antibody is shown in Fig. 3.12.3. Each antibody has several regions. The Fc region (fragment crystallizable) is the tail region and is the same for all antibodies in a class in one species. It interacts with cell surface receptors and some proteins of the complement system to activate the immune response. The Fab region contains variable sections that define the specific target antigen to which the antibody can bind.

There are five basic classes: IgA, IgG, IgM, IgD and IgE. IgA is present on mucosal surfaces to prevent infections, IgM is produced early in response to infection and IgG (of which there are three isotypes IgG_1 toIgG_3) is produced later in response to infection. IgE is thought to have a particular role in parasitic infections. The pattern of antibody production demonstrates the importance of memory in increasing the speed and strength of response with secondary exposure, and also the effect of

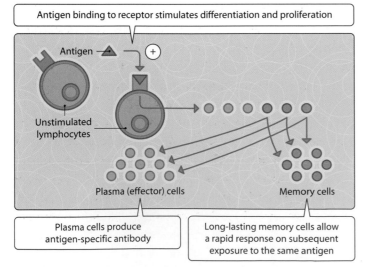

Fig. 3.12.1 Lymphocytes and immunological memory.

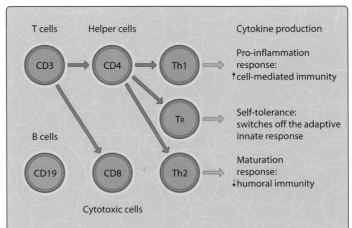

Fig. 3.12.2 The lymphocyte family.

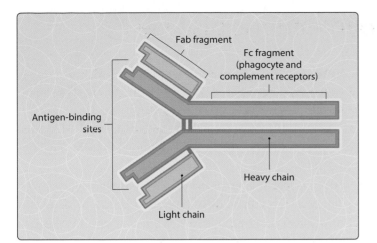

Fig. 3.12.3 Basic structure of an antibody.

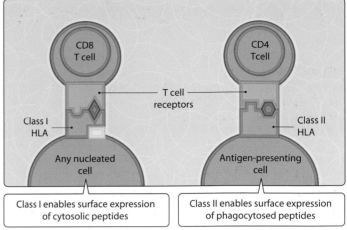

Class I enables surface expression of cytosolic peptides

Class II enables surface expression of phagocytosed peptides

Fig. 3.12.5 T cell recognition of an antigen.

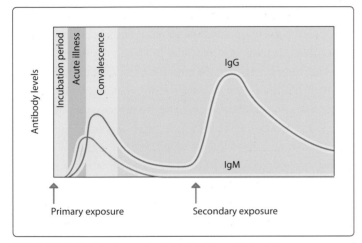

Fig. 3.12.4 Antibody production during an infection.

to antigens presented on cell surfaces and not free antigen. These antigens are presented by a type of cell surface molecule known as the **human leukocyte antigen** (**HLA**) system (which is the name of the major histocompatibility complex (MHC) in humans). There are two classes of HLA molecule. Every nucleated cell expresses a sample of its cytosolic molecules on the cell surface in association with HLA class I molecules; if the cell is manufacturing 'foreign' antigens, such as will occur in intracellular infections, particularly viral, this will be detected by **cytotoxic T cells** and they will kill the infected cell (Fig. 3.12.5).

Phagocytic cells express a sample of breakdown products from engulfed material, particularly non-viral pathogens, on their surface in association with HLA class II molecules, a set of molecules largely restricted to antigen-presenting cells. Foreign antigens will be recognized by helper T cells, whose post-activation effector cells (Th1, Th0 or Th2) produce a range of cytokines that will determine the nature of the subsequent immune response (Figs 3.12.1 and 3.12.5).

isotype switching, as IgM is only produced in primary infection (Fig. 3.12.4). Antibodies are important for:

- complement activation (initiation of the classic pathway via the Fc fragment)
- opsonization (improving the efficiency of phagocytic uptake via the Fc fragment)
- prevention of adherence (through binding to microorganism adherins)
- neutralization of toxins
- antibody-dependent cell cytotoxicity (through natural killer cell recognition of bound antibody via the Fc fragment).

T lymphocytes

T lymphocytes are important for the overall control of the immune response and for the recognition and killing of infected host cells. In contrast to B lymphocytes, they can only respond

Immune cell distribution

There is considerable movement of immune cells throughout the body. T cells mature in the thymus and B cells in the bone marrow (**primary lymphoid organs**) in the fetus, before moving to **secondary lymphoid organs**, such as the spleen, lymph nodes and mucosa-associated lymphoid tissue (MALT).

Phagocytes and debris pass from the site of infection to the secondary lymphoid organs, where lymphocyte stimulation takes place. The activated lymphocytes, and other inflammatory cells such as platelets and monocytes, are then directed back to the site of infection by activated complement factors and chemo-attractants, released by leukocytes and damaged cells at the site.

13. Upper respiratory tract infections

Questions
- What are the features of a common cold?
- How is influenza differentiated from the common cold clinically?
- What are the features of the common syndromes of upper respiratory tract infection?

The upper respiratory tract is the initial site of infection or a site of colonization for most infections of the respiratory tract (Fig. 3.13.1). It is also the site for a number of resident organisms, the prevalence of which will vary in individuals:

- common: *Streptococcus mutans* and other α-haemolytic streptococci, *Neisseria* sp., corynebacteria, *Bacteroides* spp., *Veillonella* spp., other anaerobic cocci, fusiform bacteria, *Candida albicans*, *Haemophilus influenzae*, *Entamoeba gingivalis*
- less common: *Streptococcus pyogenes*, *Streptococcus pneumoniae*, *Neisseria meningitidis*, *Staphylococcus aureus*.

Some of these resident flora can be pathogenic. Infections of the upper respiratory tract (URTIs) are the commonest acute illness. The respiratory tract has defence mechanisms that prevent infection in the normal individual (Fig. 3.13.2). The **mucociliary escalator** is the process where the mucous lining of the tract is swept upwards by the beating of cilia, thus carrying foreign particles trapped in the mucus up towards the pharynx, where it is swallowed.

Common colds/rhinitis

Children suffer two to six colds per year in industrialized countries, with this frequency halving in adulthood. This high incidence of colds is attributable to the high number of viruses and serotypes involved. Both aerosol and fomite transmission contribute to the spread of infection.

The principal findings of rhinorrhoea and sneezing are found in almost all cases. In addition, there may be sore throat, headaches and constitutional upset with fever. Earache is frequent in childhood. The diagnosis of the syndrome is clinical; laboratory identification is not required because of the current absence of appropriate antiviral therapy. Antirhinoviral therapy is, however, a possibility as drugs are developed that block the interaction between the major host cell receptor (intercellular adhesion molecule-1) and the virus receptor-binding protein in a canyon that occurs on the surface of the viral capsid. Symptomatic therapy with analgesics and decongestants is commonly employed. Vaccine development is hindered by the diverse aetiology.

Influenza

Unlike common colds, which are non-life-threatening illnesses, influenza has a significant associated mortality, particularly in the elderly and those with underlying cardiopulmonary disease. Clinically, there are three features that distinguish influenza infection from common colds: an acute onset, presence of a fever in almost all cases (occurs in the minority of common colds) and more marked constitutional upset with myalgia. Zanamivir and oseltamivir are used in the treatment and prophylaxis of

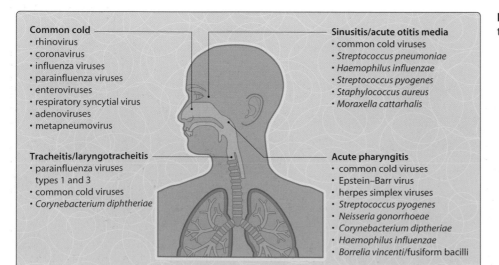

Common cold
- rhinovirus
- coronavirus
- influenza viruses
- parainfluenza viruses
- enteroviruses
- respiratory syncytial virus
- adenoviruses
- metapneumovirus

Tracheitis/laryngotracheitis
- parainfluenza viruses types 1 and 3
- common cold viruses
- *Corynebacterium diphtheriae*

Sinusitis/acute otitis media
- common cold viruses
- *Streptococcus pneumoniae*
- *Haemophilus influenzae*
- *Streptococcus pyogenes*
- *Staphylococcus aureus*
- *Moraxella cattarhalis*

Acute pharyngitis
- common cold viruses
- Epstein–Barr virus
- herpes simplex viruses
- *Streptococcus pyogenes*
- *Neisseria gonorrhoeae*
- *Corynebacterium diptheriae*
- *Haemophilus influenzae*
- *Borrelia vincenti*/fusiform bacilli

Fig. 3.13.1 Common causes of an infection of the upper respiratory tract.

influenza A infections. A vaccine is recommended for patients with underlying chronic cardiopulmonary disease, chronic renal failure or diabetes mellitus, and in the immunosuppressed. This vaccine is changed annually because the virus undergoes genetic change either through minor sequence changes (resulting in **antigenic drift**) or through recombination (resulting in **antigenic shift**), which produce changes in one or both surface proteins, the haemagglutin or neuraminidase (Fig. 3.13.3). Antigenic shift increases the likelihood of a pandemic, as even partial prior immunity to a completely new strain is absent.

Sore throat/pharyngitis and tonsillitis

Over two-thirds of sore throats are viral in aetiology and may be a continuum of infection of the nasal mucosa (common cold). *Streptococcus pyogenes* is the commonest bacterial cause and can be associated with severe complications: peritonsillar abscess, scarlet fever, rheumatic fever and acute glomeronephritis. The last two are immune-complex-mediated diseases: rheumatic fever can be systemic with myocarditis, pericarditis, polyarthritis and Sydenham's chorea.

Diphtheria

Diphtheria is caused by *Corynebacterium diphtheriae*. There is much local inflammation of the nasopharynx, with a characteristic 'bull neck' appearance from enlarged lymph nodes. Toxigenic strains of *C. diphtheriae* produce a polypeptide that causes local destruction of epithelial cells and spreads systemically to cause myocarditis and polyneuritis.

The aetiological diagnosis is made by culture of a throat swab or by serological assays. With diphtheria, toxin production should also be sought. Most viral sore throats are self-limiting and are managed symptomatically. *S. pyogenes* infections should be treated (most frequently with a penicillin) to prevent complications. Diphtheria toxin can be neutralized with antitoxin. Contacts of diphtheria should be screened and given booster vaccination and/or chemoprophylaxis as appropriate.

Sinusitis/acute otitis media

Sinusitis and acute otitis media are most frequently a complication of common colds but may also be caused by secondary bacterial invaders (Fig. 3.13.1). Localized pain is the most frequent symptom, but children with otitis media may present with unexplained fever or vomiting. If chronic infection results, surgery may be necessary in addition to antibiotics.

Epiglottitis

Epiglottitis is most commonly a disease of young children as a result of spread of bacteria from the nasopharynx. *H. influenzae* type b is the classic cause, but other bacteria may now be involved. Bacteraemia is frequent; epiglottitis may present as an acute medical emergency with respiratory obstruction. Intravenous antibiotics may be needed.

Tracheitis/laryngotracheitis

Tracheitis/laryngotracheitis causes hoarseness and retrosternal discomfort on both inspiration and expiration. Parainfluenza (and other) viruses cause swelling of the mucous membranes, which results in inspiratory stridor, termed 'croup'. Diagnosis of the specific aetiology is made by identification from a throat swab or serologically.

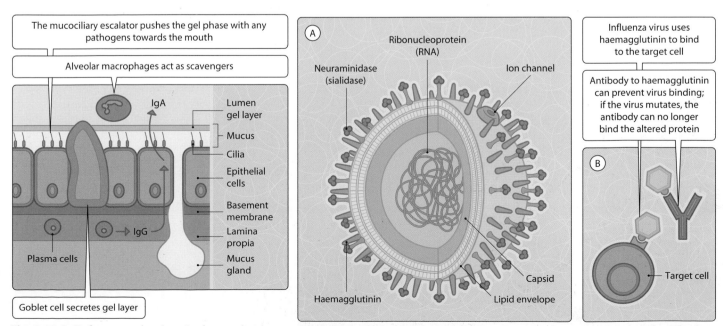

Fig. 3.13.2 Defence mechanisms in the respiratory tract.

Fig. 3.13.3 The influenza virus. A, virus structure; B, viral avoidance of antibody defences.

14. Lower respiratory tract infections

Questions
- Which lower respiratory tract infections are common?
- What are the clinical features of respiratory tract infections?
- What is the clinical management of community-acquired pneumonia?

Epidemiology

The lower respiratory tract refers to the part from the trachea to the lungs and includes the larynx. The **mucociliary escalator** (see Ch. 13) ensures that the complex and abundant bacterial flora of the upper tract is much reduced in the larynx and trachea, and the bronchi in health are sterile.

Respiratory tract infections are the most frequent cause of GP consultation, of which pneumonia only accounts for approximately 10% (Fig. 3.14.1). Patients with chronic obstructive pulmonary disease (COPD) are at risk of acute exacerbations of bacterial bronchitis when acquiring a viral infection. Respiratory syncytial virus causes **bronchiolitis** in infants who are less than 2 years of age and can cause life-threatening pneumonitis in the immunosuppressed host (e.g. transplant recipient). **Influenza** may be complicated by superinfection with bacteria, especially pneumococcal and staphylococcal pneumonia. Influenza vaccine should be given to all 'at-risk' persons in the autumn, and the drug oseltamivir is available. **Pertussis** tracheobronchitis (whooping cough) occurs in communities with low vaccination coverage, and spread may be reduced by early treatment with erythromycin. **Bacterial (typical) pneumonia** develops when bacteria overwhelm the bronchial host defences and is more common in the elderly. *Mycoplasma*, *Chlamydophila* spp.

and *Coxiella burnetii* (causes of **atypical pneumonia**) can infect the previously healthy. *Legionella pneumophila* has its reservoir in warm water and is spread by aerosol, such as those created by poorly maintained showers and air-conditioners. Typically it affects the borderline immunocompromised, for example heavy-drinking, heavy-smoking elderly persons returning from warm climates.

Coxiella sp. is a rare cause of atypical pneumonia (Q fever), affecting mainly farmers and vets (Ch. 31). **Pneumocystis jirovecii** (was *Pneumocystis carinii*) causes a bilateral pneumonia in HIV-infected patients when their CD4 cell count falls below 200 cells/µl.

In **cystic fibrosis**, the combination of thickened secretions and repeated viral, *Staphylococcus aureus* and *Haemophilus influenzae* infections in early life lead to severe bronchiectasis. Chronic infection with *Pseudomonas aeruginosa*, and sometimes *Burkholderia cepacia*, results in fatal destruction of the lung in spite of frequent courses of potent intravenous and nebulized antibiotics. However, life expectancy has increased dramatically with improved management and may do so further with gene therapy.

Aetiology and clinical features

Different organisms characteristically affect different age groups and different parts of the respiratory tract (Fig. 3.14.2), although, once infection has been initiated, the inflammation can become widespread.

In atypical pneumonia, in contrast to bacterial pneumonia, there is less production of sputum, but the systemic symptoms and chest radiography changes are greater than might be

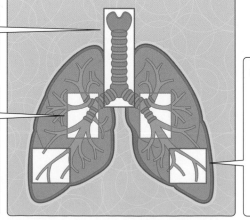

A Laryngotracheobronchitis
Inflammatory oedema causes barking cough, stridor and hoarseness
Caused by influenza, parainfluenza, adenovirus, *Bordetella pertussis*

B Bronchitis
Bronchititis is more likely in cigarette smokers or those with COPD and induces purulent sputum, rhonchi and an expiratory wheeze (bronchiolitis) but no consolidation on chest radiograph
Caused by *Streptococcus pneumoniae*, *Haemophilus influenzae*, *Moraxella catarrhalis*. Bronchiolitis is caused by respiratory syncitial virus

C Pneumonia
Inflammation of the alveoli, causing dyspnoea, fever and crepitations; consolidation is seen on chest radiograph
Bacterial pneumonia is caused by *Streptococcus pneumoniae*, *Haemophilus influenzae*, *Staphylococcus aureus*, *Pseudomonas aeruginosa*
Atypical pneumonia is caused by *Mycoplasma pneumoniae*, *Chlamydophila* spp., *Legionella pneumoniae*

Fig. 3.14.1 Respiratory tract syndromes and aetiology. A. Laryngotracheobronchitis; B. bronchitis; C. pneumonia. COPD, chronic obstructive pulmonary disease.

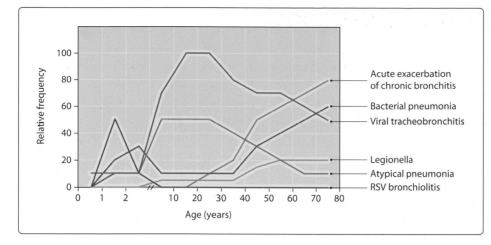

Fig. 3.14.2 Relative frequency of respiratory tract infections by age.

Acute exacerbation of chronic bronchitis

Bacterial pneumonia
Viral tracheobronchitis

Legionella
Atypical pneumonia
RSV bronchiolitis

suspected given the few signs on chest examination. Severity assessment is based on the following CURB-65 criteria:

confusion

urea > 7 mmol/l

respiratory rate > 30/min

blood pressure< 90/60 mmHg

age > **65** years.

The risk of death increases once at least two of these criteria are fulfilled, and the patient should be admitted for hospital treatment.

Hospital-acquired pneumonia is defined as a pneumonia developing at least 3 days after admission and is usually caused by multiresistant hospital bacteria such as *Pseudomonas aeruginosa*, coliforms or methicillin-resistant *S. aureus* (MRSA).

Clinical management

The great majority of infections are self-limiting, and a provisional diagnosis should be based upon the signs and symptoms (Fig. 3.14.1), with laboratory investigation confined to those that may be serious. A pernasal swab can be used for *Bordetella* culture and nasopharyngeal aspiration for respiratory viruses (Fig. 3.14.3). Sputum culture is used in suspected bacterial bronchitis and bronchopneumonia; atypical pneumonia can be investigated by urine culture for legionella antigen and serum for *Mycoplasma*, *Coxiella* and *Chlamydophila* spp.

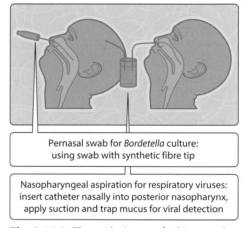

Pernasal swab for *Bordetella* culture: using swab with synthetic fibre tip

Nasopharyngeal aspiration for respiratory viruses: insert catheter nasally into posterior nasopharynx, apply suction and trap mucus for viral detection

Fig. 3.14.3 The techniques of taking swabs or nasopharyngeal aspiration for diagnosis of laryngotracheobronchitis.

Community-acquired pneumonia is treated with amoxicillin. Erythromycin should be added to cover atypical pneumonia. If more than two severity criteria are met, third-generation cephalosporins or co-amoxiclav should be given intravenously in order to cover also for the rarer aetiological agents of *H. influenzae* and *S. aureus*. Hospital-acquired pneumonia requires broad-spectrum antibiotics with activity against pseudomonas.

15. Tuberculosis and other mycobacterial diseases

Questions
- What are the clinical features of pulmonary tuberculosis?
- How is the diagnosis confirmed?
- What is the treatment and prevention of tuberculosis?
- What are the differences between lepromatous and tuberculoid leprosy?

Mycobacterium tuberculosis and *Mycobacterium leprae* are the most important mycobateria causing infections in humans, although there are a number of atypical mycobacteria that can also cause disease (Table 3.15.1).

Microbiology and pathogenesis

Mycobacteria are thin rods with a very different cell wall structure compared with other bacteria. The high lipid and mycolic acid content in the cell wall resists conventional Gram staining and special stains such as the acid- and alcohol-based Ziehl–Neelsen stain is required to make them visible under the microscope (see Fig. 3.3.4A). Based on this stain, the bacteria are also known as acid-fast bacilli (AFB). Most mycobacteria are slow growing (up to 6 weeks) and require special culture medium (e.g. Lowenstein–Jensen agar).

Mycobacteria are intracellular organisms that survive and multiply in macrophages. Intact cell-mediated immunity helps to wall off the bacteria in infected tissues by forming granulomas

Table 3.15.1 CLASSIFICATION OF MYCOBACTERIA

Species	Source	Disease
M. tuberculosis complex		
M. tuberculosis	Human	Tuberculosis
M. bovis	Animals	Tuberculosis
M. africanum	Human	Tuberculosis
M. microti	Animals	Tuberculosis
M. leprae	Human	Leprosy (Hansen's disease)
Atypical mycobacteria (non-tuberculous mycobacteria)		
M. avium–intra-cellulare	Birds	Pneumonia, diarrhoea in the immunosuppressed
M. kansasii	Environment	Pneumonia in the immunosuppressed
M. marinum	Fresh water	Skin granuloma
M. ulcerans	Environment	Buruli ulcer (Africa)

(also called **tubercle**). Mycobacteria can lay dormant for many years until they are reactivated. This may occur if the patient's cellular immune system is compromised, such as in old age, corticosteroid use or HIV infection.

Epidemiology and clinical manifestation of tuberculosis

One third of the world population is infected with tuberculosis (TB) and the disease kills around 5000 people a day. TB is endemic in countries, which have under-funded public healthcare (Fig. 3.15.1). HIV coinfections are common in places such as sub-Saharan Africa and are associated with a higher mortality. The bacteria are transmitted via air-borne droplet nuclei from human to human. The first exposure often leads to subclinical (asymptomatic) primary infection, although a proportion of infected individuals progress to active disease, usually affecting the lungs (Fig. 3.15.2). Secondary or reactivated TB occurs most commonly in the lungs and patients present with:

- low-grade fever
- night sweats
- weight loss
- blood-stained productive cough (haematemesis).

TB can also affect many extrapulmonary sites, such as the CNS, causing tuberculous meningitis; the kidneys, presenting with sterile pyuria (characterized by pus cells seen in urine microscopy without 'bacterial' growth); and bone and joints, causing destruction of vertebrae or chronic arthritis. Disseminated TB (referred to as miliary TB) can affect multiple organs including the lungs, which show a millet-seed type pattern in radiographs.

Diagnosis, treatment and prevention

The diagnosis is made on the basis of typical signs and symptoms and is confirmed by positive microbiology. A saline-induced sputum from a symptomatic patient with pulmonary TB is often positive by Ziehl–Neelsen stain (Fig. 3.15.3) but the microscopy does not differentiate TB from other *Mycobacteria* species. Speciation and drug-susceptibility testing is achieved by using specific culture methods. An urgent confirmation of the diagnosis and speciation may also be obtained by rapid testing of patient specimens using molecular techniques. Such tests can also be used to detect mutations in bacterial genes that are associated with antibiotic resistance e.g. *rpoB* mutations conferring rifampicin resistance.

Skin testing with the **Mantoux test** (intradermal injection of a purified *M. tuberculosis* protein derivative) may be another option to confirm exposure to TB, but this test may also be

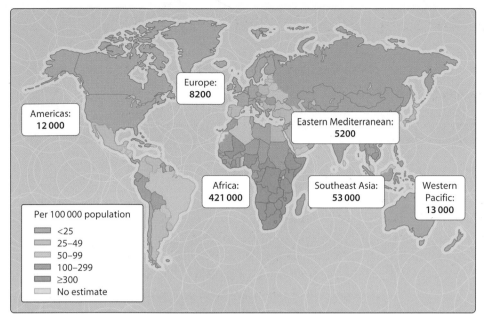

Fig. 3.15.1 Worldwide distribution of tuberculosis.

Europe:
8200

Americas:
12 000

Eastern Mediterranean:
5200

Africa:
421 000

Southeast Asia:
53 000

Western Pacific:
13 000

Per 100 000 population
<25
25–49
50–99
100–299
≥300
No estimate

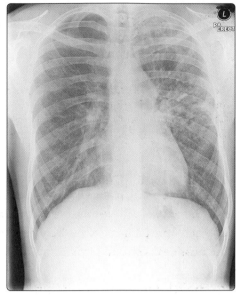

Fig. 3.15.2 Primary tuberculosis. Chest radiograph showing miliary lesions in left upper lobe.

positive in individuals vaccinated with BCG (Bacille Calmette-Guérin). More specific is the in vitro detection of interferon-γ from macrophages after exposure to TB-specific antigens.

If left untreated, the natural progression of the infection results in death in 50%, in spontaneous recovery in 25% while 25% remain infectious. TB is, therefore, treated with multiple antibiotics for prolonged periods of time to prevent treatment failures and also to avoid **drug resistance** developing. The first-line treatment of pulmonary infection is usually for 2 months with four drugs (rifampicin, isoniazid, pyrazinamide and ethambutol or streptomycin) followed by 4 months with two drugs (rifampicin and isoniazid). The treatment of multidrug-resistant TB is a difficult clinical challenge as the bacteria may be resistant to many first-line antibiotics (e.g. rifampicin, isoniazid) and other more toxic second-line drugs (ethionamide, ciprofloxacin, amikacin, cycloserine) may need to be used.

Patients with pulmonary TB are infectious and should be placed in negative pressure isolation if they are admitted into the hospital. Staff should wear protective clothing including special face masks to minimize the risk of transmission. It is the role of the public health officer to trace people in the community that have had contact with someone with known pulmonary TB so that they can receive prophylactic antibiotics or be monitored for the infection.

Epidemiology and management of *leprosy*

There are 5.5 million people affected by leprosy, in particularly in the endemic areas in India, Mexico, Africa and the Pacific Islands. Infection requires prolonged close contact with an infected patient. The diagnosis is made clinically in conjunction with a skin biopsy, which may show mycobacteria in the histology.

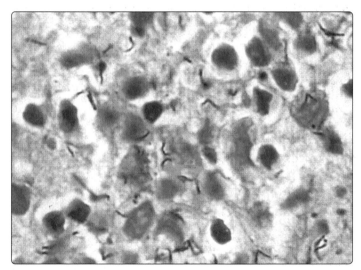

Fig. 3.15.3 Ziehl–Neelsen stain for mycobacteria in sputum.

Unlike *M. tuberculosis*, *M. leprae* can only be cultured in certain animals and not in artificial culture medium. Clinically there are two forms of the infection:

Lepromatous leprosy. This form occurs in patients who cannot mount a good immune response. They develop many skin lesions, destruction of nasal cartilage (saddle nose) and peripheral nerve thickening, leading to loss of sensation and deformation of toes and fingers. Numerous mycobacteria are found in skin biopsy.

Tuberculoid leprosy. Patients who can mount a good cell-mediated immune response have fewer skin lesions with no mycobacteria in the skin biopsy.

Treatment of leprosy includes the use of dapsone, rifampin and clofazimine.

16. Meningitis

Questions
- What are the characteristic cerebrospinal fluid findings in bacterial meningitis?
- Which causes of viral meningitis are common?
- How can the spread of meningococcus be controlled in a community?

Infection of the meninges follows invasion across the blood–brain or blood–cerebrospinal fluid (CSF) barrier. Organisms may, rarely, gain direct access following surgery, trauma or (in amoebic infections) directly through the cribriform plate.

Viral meningitis
Most infections are acute and the commonest pathogens are viruses, especially in children and young adults. Patients with viral meningitis often present with an influenza-like illness with headache, sore throat and muscle pains. The features of meningitis then follow but tend to be milder than in bacterial infections and less rapid in onset. The common causes are the herpesviruses (family Herpesviridae) herpes simplex virus (HSV), varicella zoster virus and Epstein–Barr virus; the enteroviruses (family Picornaviridae) echovirus, coxsackievirus and mumps virus; and the Flaviviridae family, which includes West Nile virus and Japanese encephalitis virus.

Most viral meningitis resolves completely without specific treatment. However HSV meningitis, which occurs after primary HSV2 infections or in HSV reactivations in the immunosuppressed and elderly, requires intravenous aciclovir treatment.

Enteroviruses, HSV and mumps are common causes of viral meningitis. The most prominent manifestation of mumps is, however, parotitis. Epididymo-orchitis may, uncommonly, result in sterility; thyroiditis, pancreatitis, meningo-encephalitis, myocarditis and arthritis are rare complications.

Bacterial meningitis
In contrast to viral forms, bacterial meningitis may be life threatening and have serious sequelae for those who survive. While it may be impossible to predict the causative agent from the clinical features, some pathogens are more common at certain ages (Fig. 3.16.1). Neonatal meningitis may be early (within 7 days of birth) or late (occurring between 1 week and 3 months) onset. Early infections are acquired from the mother, whereas late infections may result from cross-infection after birth. The commonest causes of early-onset disease are group B β-haemolytic streptococci and coliforms such as *Escherichia coli*. *Listeria*

monocytogenes and group B β-haemolytic streptococci can cause late-onset disease. Most bacterial meningitis occurs in childhood. The introduction of Hib vaccine against type B strains of *Haemophilus influenzae* has significantly reduced the incidence of invasive infections caused by this organism. The commonest cause is now *Neisseria meningitidis*. The three common serotypes A, B and C vary in prevalence, but B and C are commonest in western Europe and A in Arabic countries. The introduction of conjugated meningococcal C vaccine in the UK significantly reduced the incidence of meningococcal meningitis. Meningitis caused by *Streptococcus pneumoniae* occurs at all ages but particularly in children under 2 years, the elderly and those with immune defects (e.g. HIV infection, sickle-cell disease and post-splenectomy). Meningitis in adolescents and young adults is most commonly caused by meningococci. In later life, pneumococci are more likely. *L. monocytogenes* is a relatively rare cause but should be considered particularly in pregnant and immunocompromised patients. Tuberculous meningitis occurs more commonly in immigrants from developing countries.

Clinical features of meningitis
The characteristic clinical features of meningitis are:
- headache
- irritability or drowsiness, sometimes with alteration of consciousness
- fever
- neck stiffness
- photophobia
- Positive Kernig's sign (pain in the lumbar region on straight-leg raising).

Acute meningococcal disease may present as a septicaemic illness without meningitis. Such infections are often characterized by a petechial rash, and patients may develop endotoxin shock. In contrast, the onset of TB meningitis is often gradual with days or weeks of general malaise before the onset of meningeal features. Diagnosis may be difficult in the early stages, but localizing neurological signs such as cranial nerve palsies are helpful.

Diagnosis
Blood cultures should always be taken, preferably before antibiotics are started. Examination of CSF is advisable whenever possible. Patients at risk of raised intracranial pressure (focal neurological deficits, known immunosuppression or mass lesions) should undergo computed tomography or magnetic resonance imaging before lumbar puncture. The CSF is examined for the presence and type of white blood cells

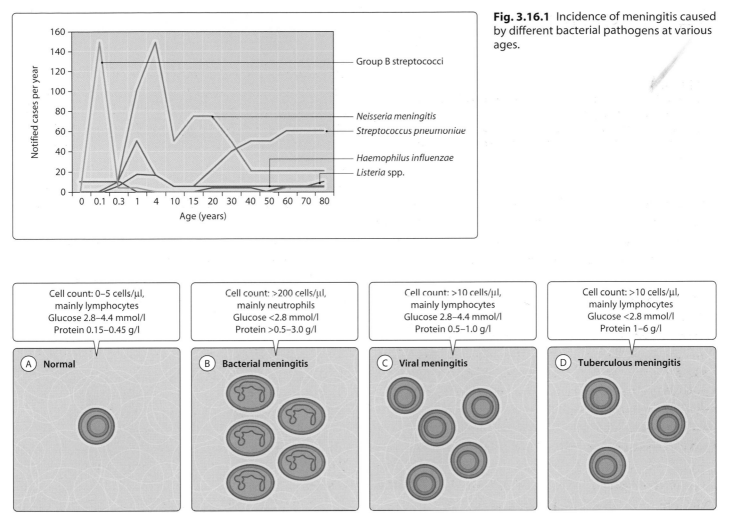

Fig. 3.16.1 Incidence of meningitis caused by different bacterial pathogens at various ages.

Group B streptococci

Neisseria meningitis
Streptococcus pneumoniae

Haemophilus influenzae
Listeria spp.

A Normal	B Bacterial meningitis	C Viral meningitis	D Tuberculous meningitis
Cell count: 0–5 cells/μl, mainly lymphocytes Glucose 2.8–4.4 mmol/l Protein 0.15–0.45 g/l	Cell count: >200 cells/μl, mainly neutrophils Glucose <2.8 mmol/l Protein >0.5–3.0 g/l	Cell count: >10 cells/μl, mainly lymphocytes Glucose 2.8–4.4 mmol/l Protein 0.5–1.0 g/l	Cell count: >10 cells/μl, mainly lymphocytes Glucose <2.8 mmol/l Protein 1–6 g/l

Fig. 3.16.2 Typical cerebrospinal fluid white cell findings in meningitis.

(Fig. 3.16.2), red blood cells, protein content and glucose level (Table 3.16.1). Additional investigations should include the following, particularly if the patient has already received antibiotics:

- throat swab for meningococcal culture
- blood for meningococcal polymerase chain reaction (PCR)
- acute serum for meningococcal antibodies and antigen detection.

Treatment and prophylaxis of bacterial meningitis

Treatment must be prompt, and immediate parenteral penicillin (before hospital admission) is recommended in suspected meningococcal disease. Ceftriaxone or cefotaxime are first choice for empirical treatment. *Listeria* spp. are resistant to cephalosporin, and amoxicillin should be added if this is suspected. In neonates, addition of gentamicin covers for coliforms. Concomitant steroid therapy has been shown to be beneficial for *H. influenzae* type B and pneumococcal meningitis.

Table 3.16.1 CEREBROSPINAL FLUID FINDINGS IN MENINGITIS

	Pressure (mmHg)	Glucose (mmol/l)[a]	Protein (g/l)
Normal	100–200	2.8–4.4	0.15–0.45
Acute bacterial	Raised	Very reduced	0.5–3.0
Viral	Normal or raised	Normal	0.5–1.0
Tuberculous	Normal or raised	Reduced	1.0–6.0

[a]The ratio of CSF/blood for glucose is more important than the absolute level of glucose: the normal CSF glucose is approximately 60% of that in blood.

Chemoprophylaxis of close contacts is recommended in meningococcal (and *H. influenzae*) disease to reduce the risk of secondary cases. In addition, contacts of cases of serotypes A and C meningococcal disease may be vaccinated—a reliable type B vaccine is still awaited. Patients over 2 years of age at increased risk of pneumococcal disease should be immunized with a polyvalent vaccine.

17. Encephalitis and other nervous system infections

Questions
- What are the causes of encephalitis?
- What are the different types of myelitis?
- What are the features of brain abscess?
- What are the different types of neuritis?

Infections occur in the brain (**encephalitis** and **brain abscess**), spinal cord (**myelitis**), nerves (**neuritis** or **polyneuritis**), or a combination of these. The nervous system is normally sterile, and infections either have to traverse the blood–brain barrier or be directly inoculated. Unlike meningitis, which often recovers without sequelae, nervous tissue has poor repair mechanisms, and tissue damage leads to long-term sequelae.

Encephalitis
Encephalitis is predominantly a viral disease (Table 3.17.1), with herpes simplex infection being the most common in the UK (Fig. 3.17.1). Cerebral dysfunction presents as behavioural disturbance, fits and diminished consciousness. If progressive, then localized neurological signs, coma and death may occur. Diagnosis of the condition is clinical with confirmation from imaging and electroencephalography. Virus may also be detectable in the cerebrospinal fluid (CSF) but may not be cultivable. Brain biopsy offers the definitive means of diagnosis but is only used in specialist centres. Herpes simplex virus (HSV) encephalitis has a 70% mortality unless treated with aciclovir. Rabies is fatal but can be treated with postexposure prophylaxis, as the long incubation period allows time for an adequate immune response.

Brain abscess
Brain abscesses are predominantly bacterial in origin and arise because of spread from other sites such as infected cardiac valves and bones, mastoid sinuses and chronic middle ear infection. Pathogens include *Staphylococcus aureus*, streptococci, Gram-negative bacilli and anaerobes, and infections are often mixed. Localized neurological signs are common. Multiple abscesses/cysts may be caused by bacteria, or the zoonoses hydatid disease (*Echinococcus granulosus*), toxocariasis (*Toxocara* spp.) or cysticercosis (tapeworm). Diagnosis is by imaging and, for the helminth diseases, by serology. Single abscesses are treated empirically with antibiotics such as ceftriaxone and metronidazole, usually in conjunction with surgical drainage. Appropriate chemotherapy is used for helminth infections, with consideration of poor transfer of most antimicrobial drugs across the non-inflamed blood–brain barrier.

Table 3.17.1 CAUSES OF ENCEPHALITIS

Cause	Features
Viruses	
Herpes simplex virus (herpesvirus)	Bitemporal localization detectable by imaging; HSV2 common in neonates, HSV2 in adults
Mumps virus (herpesvirus)	Meningoencephalitis may precede parotitis
Eastern and Western equine encephalitis virus (toga/bunyavirus)	Mosquito-borne in parts of North America
Rabies virus (rhabdovirus)	Incubation period of weeks to months after mammal bite; fatal if not treated
Tick-borne flaviviruses	Forested areas of Scandinavia; vaccine available
Japanese B virus (flavivirus)	Southeast Asia; vaccine available
Poliovirus and enteroviruses	Most commonly causes meningitis but may cause meningoencephalitis
Rubella and measles viruses	Subacute panencephalitis with high mortality
JC virus (papovavirus)	Progressive multifocal leukoencephalopathy in the immunocompromised
Post-viral infection/post-vaccination	Immune mediated; occurs with measles, influenza and others; good prognosis
Protozoa/fungi	
Toxoplasma gondii	Immunocompromised and newborn
Cryptococcus neoformans	Common in HIV infection
Plasmodium falciparum	Cerebral malaria
Trypanosomas spp.	Sleeping sickness; central Africa
Prions	Creutzfeldt–Jakob disease

Myelitis
Myelitis may accompany encephalitis (**encephalomyelitis**) but may present as the predominant feature. **Poliomyelitis** is an infection of the anterior horn cells and motor neurons with poliovirus or other enteroviruses, causing a flaccid paralysis that may lead to residual muscle wasting from disuse; paralytic poliomyelitis occurs, however, in fewer than 1% of poliovirus

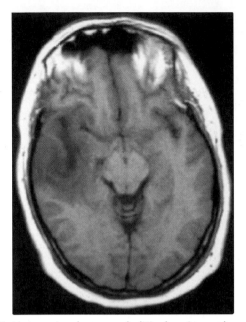

Fig. 3.17.1 Herpes simplex encephalitis showing oedema in the right temporal lobe.

infections. Rabies may cause an ascending flaccid paralysis if bites occur on the lower extremities.

Transverse myelitis with bilateral flaccid or spastic paraparesis now occurs more commonly with other infectious agents as poliovirus vaccination is implemented worldwide:

- postinfectious myelitis: influenza and other upper respiratory tract infections, measles, rubella, mumps, vaccines
- direct infection of the spinal cord: varicella zoster virus, human T cell lymphotropic virus, *Borrelia burgdoferi* (Lyme disease)
- vasculitis of the anterior spinal artery: *Mycobacterium tuberculosis*, *Treponema pallidum* (syphilis), schistosomiasis.

Neuritis/polyneuritis

Direct infection of nerves with Schwann cell degeneration, which may be followed by axonal degeneration, results from infections with *Mycobacterium leprae*, *Trypanosoma* spp., microsporidia and cytomegalovirus. Flaccid paralysis results. Varicella zoster virus causes the Ramsay–Hunt syndrome, which presents with vesicles in the ear canal and a unilateral facial nerve palsy.

Infections such as tetanus, botulism and diphtheria produce **neurotoxins**, which interfere with synaptic transmission.

Guillain–Barré syndrome is an ascending bilateral paralysis that is generally preceded by an infection up to 4 weeks prior to onset. Campylobacter gastroenteritis is the commonest precipitant, but other gastrointestinal and respiratory tract infective causes have also been noted. An autoimmune aetiology is postulated.

Bell's palsy, a normally transient unilateral facial palsy, may be aetiologically associated with herpes simplex infection, although there is little benefit from the use of aciclovir.

CASE STUDY: Encephalitis

JV is a 35-year-old office worker who was brought to the emergency department of his local hospital because he was becoming increasingly confused and disoriented over a period of 2 days. He was awake but drowsy on arrival and it was difficult to get a history from him, but his wife reported that he had been previously well and was not on medication. His only complaint was that he has had a 'bit of a headache' over the last few days. Apart from a fever of 38.1°C and the drowsiness, examination revealed no abnormalities, and specifically there were no focal neurological signs. In the absence of papilloedema, he had a lumbar puncture and a magnetic resonance imaging (MRI) scan. His lumbar puncture showed slightly bloodstained fluid with leucocytes $120 \times 10^9/l$, 75% lymphocytes, glucose (CSF) 3.5 mmol/l (blood glucose 5.1 mmol/l) and protein 1.8 g/l. No organisms were detected. The MRI showed focal areas of attenuation in the temporal lobes. A probable diagnosis of herpes simplex encephalitis was made and he was treated with acyclovir. This was subsequently confirmed by polymerase chain reaction (PCR) but not by culture.

Viral encephalitis most frequently manifests with fever and non-specific neurological features. The commonest cause is herpes simplex regardless of whether the patient has a past history of herpes simplex infections. In this centre, MRI is now routinely used to detect the characteristic temporal lobe changes as it is more sensitive than computed tomography. PCR is also more sensitive than culture, the latter more commonly than not being negative.

18. Eye infections

Questions
■ What is the difference between exogenous and endogenous endophthalmitis?
■ What factors contribute to the development of conjunctivitis?

Ocular defence mechanisms

The eye is normally well protected against infections (Fig. 3.18.1). Physical factors such as the blinking action of the eyelid, the tear film and the conjunctiva help to prevent attachment of microorganisms. The outer eye contains antimicrobial compounds produced by the tear film (Fig.3.18.2) and phagocytic by conjunctival epithelial cells and polymorphonuclear leukocytes.

A variety of different pathogens affect different anatomical structures, resulting in disease of varying severity, ranging from relative common and less severe (e.g. stye) to permanent loss of visual acuity or even blindness (retinochoroiditis). There are two main routes of infection. The most common is direct inoculation of pathogens into the eye (exogenous infections) through trauma (i.e. surgery, foreign body, contact lenses). The second route is much rarer and introduces pathogens into the posterior part of the eye (retina/choroids) via the bloodstream (endogenous infection) (Fig.3.18.1).

Infections of the external eye structures

Infections of the ocular soft tissue around the eye can present as a painful, red swelling (**orbital cellulitis**). The infection is rare and may derive from the parasinuses or following haematogenous spread of organisms. *Streptococcus pneumoniae*, *Haemophilus influenzae* and *Staphylococcus aureus* are often the cause and may be recovered from blood cultures; eye swabs are rarely useful. In many cases, empirical antibiotic treatment is initiated prior to any positive culture. If the infection is left untreated, it can progress into serious conditions such as subperiosteal abscess or life-threatening cavernous sinus thrombosis.

The eyelid is a common site of infection, affecting the lid margins (**blepharitis**) or its sebaceous glands (meibomian glands), causing a painful swelling (**stye**). Bacteria such as staphylococci are a common cause of this infection.

Conjunctivitis is a relatively common infection caused by bacteria (e.g. *Chlamydia* sp., *S. pneumoniae*, *H. influenzae*) or viruses (e.g. adenovirus, enterovirus). Symptoms are intense hyperaemia of the conjunctival vessels ('red eye'), excessive discharge and a 'gritty' sensation in the eye. The discharge caused by bacterial conjunctivitis is thick and purulent, resulting in a 'sticky eye', whereas viral conjunctivitis presents with a watery discharge, often in both eyes. In some generalized viral infections such as measles, conjunctivitis is common. Some viral infections (particularly those caused by adenovirus) spread easily from person to person or through poorly disinfected ophthalmological equipment or shared eye protectors (shipyard eye).

Neonatal conjunctivitis caused by *Neisseria gonorrhoeae* (**ophthalmia neonatorum**) and *Chlamydia trachomatis* serotypes D–K (**inclusion conjunctivitis**) are serious conditions acquired

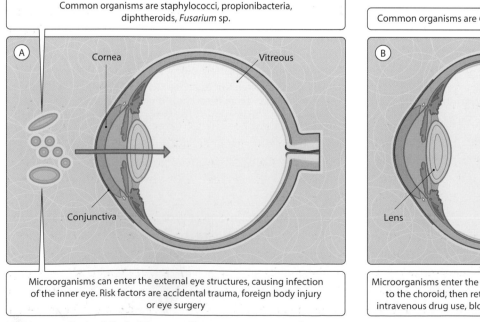

Common organisms are staphylococci, propionibacteria, diphtheroids, *Fusarium* sp.

A — Cornea — Vitreous — Conjunctiva

Microorganisms can enter the external eye structures, causing infection of the inner eye. Risk factors are accidental trauma, foreign body injury or eye surgery

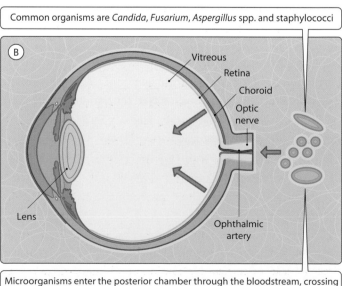

Common organisms are *Candida*, *Fusarium*, *Aspergillus* spp. and staphylococci

B — Vitreous — Retina — Choroid — Optic nerve — Lens — Ophthalmic artery

Microorganisms enter the posterior chamber through the bloodstream, crossing to the choroid, then retina and enter the vitreous humour. Risk factors are intravenous drug use, bloodstream infections, surgery or immunosuppression

Fig. 3.18.1 Endophthalmitis caused by exogenous or endogenous sources.

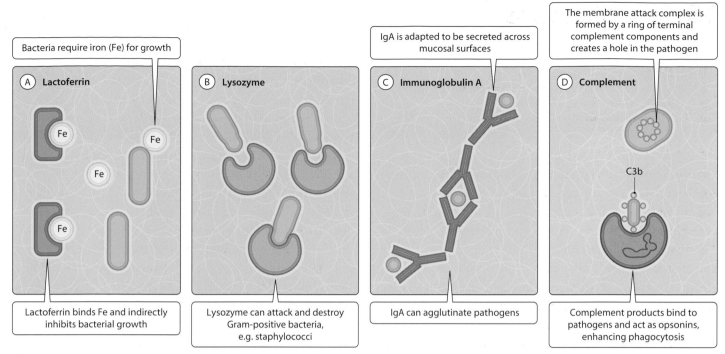

Fig. 3.18.2 Antimicrobial components of tears.

from the female genital tract during birth. It can progress to keratitis, perforation and blindness. **Trachoma** is a severe *C. trachomatis* serotype A–C infection commonly found in the tropics in all age groups. Patients present with chronic inflammation of the conjunctival epithelium, which can lead to intense scarring and blindness. Early treatment with tetracycline in adults or erythromycin in children and pregnancy is essential.

Intraocular infections

Corneal infection (**keratitis**) can be by viruses, bacteria, fungi or protozoa. Reactivation of dormant herpes simplex from the trigeminal ganglion is the most common viral keratitis, presenting as a branching, dendritic ulcer. Bacterial keratitis is often caused by *S. pneumoniae* and staphylococci. Patients present with pain, photophobia and increased tear production. The infection usually arises from direct injury to the cornea or following eye surgery. Contaminated contact lenses may also cause keratitis from the water-borne bacterium *Pseudomonas aeruginosa* or the soil and water amoeba *Acanthamoeba*. Fungal keratitis (e.g. *Fusarium* sp.) is more common in hot humid climates.

Keratitis presents with a painful corneal stromal infiltrate or central abscess with overlying epithelial defect. The resulting ulcer can lead to corneal perforation and blindness. Crescent-shaped pus may accumulate in the **anterior chamber** (the aqueous humour-filled space between the cornea, iris and lense) of the eye, also known as **hypopyon**. Keratitis is a serious infection,

requiring prompt diagnosis, intensive antimicrobial therapy and possibly corneal grafting. Prion diseases can be transmitted through corneal transplantation.

Endophthalmitis involves inflammation of the intraocular cavities (i.e. the aqueous or vitreous humours). In exogenous infections, microorganisms enter the eye through external inoculation after eye surgery (e.g. cataract) or through accidental trauma; in endogenous infections they enter the posterior part of the eye via the bloodstream from other sites of infection. Bacterial flora from the eyelid and conjunctival sac are the common organisms causing postsurgical infections, although environmental fungi (*Fusarium* sp.) may also be important in trauma. In the rarer endogenous endophthalmitis, the bacteria (e.g. *S. aureus*) or fungi (*Candida, Aspergillus* spp.) can be lodged in the highly vascularized chorioretino plexus. This haematogenous spread is rare but can potentially lead to blindness and may necessitate surgical removal of the eye (enucleation). Early diagnosis and prompt intravitreal and systemic antimicrobial therapy are vital in the successful treatment of this condition.

Unlike the rest of the eye, the **retina** and **choroid** have a rich vascular supply and blood-borne microorganisms can cause **retinochoroiditis**. Parasites (e.g. *Onchocerca volvulus* river blindness), *Toxoplasma gondii* and *Toxocara canis*), fungi (e.g. *Candida, Aspergillus* spp.) and viruses (e.g. cytomegalovirus reactivation in AIDS) are well-recognized causes. The condition is extremely difficult to treat and may result in blindness.

19. Viral skin rashes

Questions
- What are the general features of rashes caused by viruses?
- Compare an enanthem and exanthem
- What are the causes of viral skin rashes?

Viruses cause rashes with four basic components (Fig. 3.19.1):
- macular/maculopapular
- vesicular/pustular
- papular/nodular
- haemorrhagic/petechial.

Enteroviruses cause rashes of any type, including vesicular rashes with a zosteriform distribution. The cause of the cutaneous eruption is not necessarily direct virus infection.

Macular/maculopapular rashes

The macular/maculopapular rashes are most common in childhood and are not true infections of the skin. Rather they are **exanthems** (Fig. 3. 19.2), the primary infection occurring elsewhere with the rash as a secondary, probably immune-mediated, phenomenon. The virus cannot be easily, if at all, isolated from the rash. An **enanthem** (Fig. 3. 19.3), a rash on a mucous membrane, may also be detectable early in the illness; in measles these are called Koplik's spots and manifest as white flecks on the buccal mucosa. Transmission is by the respiratory route, with upper respiratory tract symptoms being common, if transient.

Measles, a paramyxovirus, can cause a severe infection with constitutional symptoms and marked upper respiratory tract symptoms. It may be complicated by secondary bacterial pneumonia, typically from *Staphylococcus aureus*. It may also be complicated by neurological disease: acute 'postinfectious' measles encephalitis, which is immune mediated; subacute encephalitis, which can occur in immunocompromised patients; and, rarely, subacute sclerosing

panencephalitis, occurring 5–10 years after primary infection. In children, particularly those with protein malnutrition, measles remains a common cause of death in the developing world.

Rubella classically manifests as a rash that starts on the face then spreads to the trunk with lymphadenopathy. It may be complicated by encephalitis, haematological deficiencies and an arthritis that affects small and medium-sized joints. The most serious manifestation, however, occurs if a pregnant woman is infected: the **congenital rubella syndrome** causes neural, cardiac, bone and other abnormalities in the fetus.

Other common causes of a maculopapular rash are parvovirus B19, which results in erythema infectiosum and human herpesvirus 6 (HHV6), which is associated with roseola infantum. Erythema infectiosum is commonly known as 'slapped cheek syndome' as the facial rash has that appearance. It is often complicated by a painful arthropathy in adults and may precipitate fetal loss in second trimester pregnancy and aplastic crises in those with haemolytic anaemia. Roseola infantum classically is preceded by 3–5 days of fever, which then leads to a rash on the trunk that spreads centrifugally.

Diagnosis

Confirmation of a clinical diagnosis is not usually required but can be made by culture of the virus from the respiratory tract or urine (measles and rubella), or serologically (rubella, B19, HHV6). Management of cases is symptomatic unless complicated. The measles–mumps–rubella vaccine (MMR) should be given in early childhood.

Vesicular/pustular rashes

The common vesicular/vesicopustular rashes are chickenpox, herpes, and hand, foot and mouth syndrome. Smallpox resembled chickenpox but has now been officially eradicated from the community.

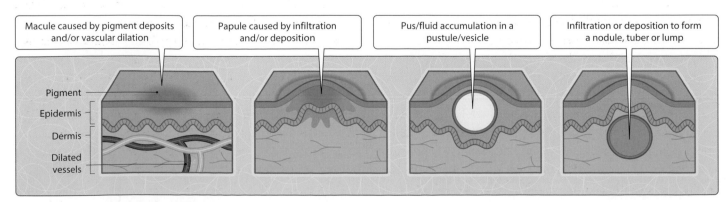

| Macule caused by pigment deposits and/or vascular dilation | Papule caused by infiltration and/or deposition | Pus/fluid accumulation in a pustule/vesicle | Infiltration or deposition to form a nodule, tuber or lump |

Pigment
Epidermis
Dermis
Dilated vessels

Fig. 3.19.1 Components of a viral rash.

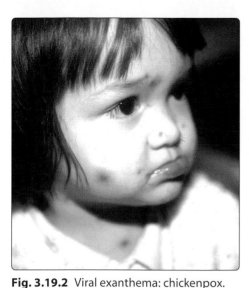

Fig. 3.19.2 Viral exanthema: chickenpox.

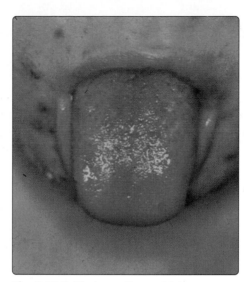

Fig. 3.19.3 Viral enanthem: chickenpox.

Diagnosis and treatment

Diagnosis of these infections is clinical, although VZV and HSV infection can be confirmed serologically. Aciclovir and derivatives are used in potentially complicated herpesvirus (VZV and HSV) infections, including ophthalmic infection.

Papular/nodular rashes

Common papulonodular rashes are warts and molluscum contagiosum. The former are caused by human papillomaviruses (HPV) and the latter by a virus of the same name. They are usually both multiple, with the distinguishing feature of molluscum contagiosum being a central umbilicus in the nodule.

The causes of these rashes are common, infectious and, usually, not life threatening. The exception is specific types of HPV (mainly types 16 and 18), which are associated with cervical cancer. Diagnosis is clinical, and treatment is by physical methods such as freezing, chemicals or surgery (if warts are large). Interferon can be injected into warts.

Haemorrhagic/petechial rashes

Some viruses uncommonly cause thrombocytopenia, manifesting as petechiae or, less frequently, haemorrhage: Epstein–Barr virus, rubella virus, cytomegalovirus, parvovirus B19, HIV, VZV and measles virus. Other clinical manifestations are usually present.

Some tropical haemorrhagic fever viruses produce widespread haemorrhage into the skin and organs by disseminated intravascular coagulation; this results in thromboses, infarcts and increased vascular permeability. There are many types distributed around the world, with Lassa, Marburg, Ebola, dengue and yellow fever being the best studied and most prevalent. Diagnosis is made by the clinical history including geography of travel and confirmed by serology. Lassa fever is treatable with ribavirin.

Mucocutaneous lymph node syndrome (**Kawasaki disease**) is an acute febrile illness of children which is caused by widespread vasculitis. Its aetiology is thought to be microbial. The manifestations are conjunctivitis, desquamative erythema affecting the mouth, tongue, hands and feet, and lymphadenopathy. There is a high 'complication' rate, with arthralgia, obstructive jaundice and life-threatening myocarditis. Clinical diagnosis, accompanied by electrocardiography, should be prompt so that treatment can be instituted with immunoglobulin and antiplatelet therapy.

Chickenpox, caused by varicella zoster virus (VZV), is spread by the respiratory route, with an exanthem and enanthem. The exanthema appears initially on the trunk, classically as crops of macules that become vesicles then pustules. At any one time, several stages can be seen, and there is usually associated pruritus. Infection may be complicated by pneumonia, Reyes' syndrome, encephalitis and secondary bacterial infection. Recurrence of chickenpox is rare.

Herpes zoster is caused by reactivation of dormant virus. Initial acquisition of virus can allow dormancy in the dorsal ganglia. Subsequent reduced cell-mediated immunity (e.g. in the elderly, in cancer patients or with immunosuppressive therapy) allows the virus to track down the sensory nerve to cause a rash in the supplied dermatome. Herpes zoster may result in neuralgia, and if ophthalmic can result in corneal scarring.

Herpes infection, with herpes simplex virus (HSV), manifests as multiple painful vesicles without cropping. Infections recur but primary infections tend to be most severe with constitutional upset. HSV, like VZV, exhibits latency in ganglia, with recurrence in the skin of the supplied nerve. HSV2 has a higher recurrence rate than HSV1.

Hand, foot and mouth disease is caused by coxsackievirus A and other enteroviruses; there are vesicles, mainly on the buccal mucosa, tongue and interdigitally on the hands and feet.

The vesicles in these infections contain virus, and transmissibility is high to susceptible individuals such as the immunocompromised and newborn. Hand, foot and mouth disease is not severe, but herpesvirus infections may become disseminated, with organ damage and possible death. Infection control measures should be considered and exposed susceptible individuals managed with antiviral drugs and/or, in the case of VZV infection, zoster immunoglobulin.

20. Bacterial and fungal skin infections

Questions
- What are the common risk factors for bacterial and fungal skin infections?
- What are the common bacteria causing skin infections and how does each present clinically?

Pathogenesis and risk factors

The skin provides an important physical barrier to infection. The normal commensal flora helps to prevent the multiplication and invasion of pathogens. Infections of the skin and deeper tissues often follow trauma, surgery or burns but may arise following even minor damage to the epidermis. Patients who have an impaired immune system (e.g. diabetes mellitus, steroid use, AIDS) are at greater risk of infection.

Some infections involve only the superficial structures of the skin, while others affect the deeper soft tissues below the dermis (Fig. 3.20.1). The infection may be localized or spreading depending on the tissue plane involved and the virulence of the pathogen.

Bacterial super-infections may complicate skin disorders such as eczema. In addition some systemic infections also present with skin features (Fig. 3.20.2).

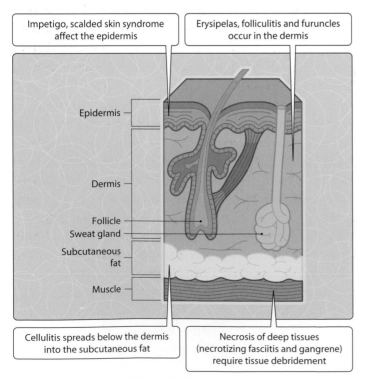

Impetigo, scalded skin syndrome affect the epidermis

Erysipelas, folliculitis and furuncles occur in the dermis

Epidermis

Dermis

Follicle
Sweat gland
Subcutaneous fat

Muscle

Cellulitis spreads below the dermis into the subcutaneous fat

Necrosis of deep tissues (necrotizing fasciitis and gangrene) require tissue debridement

Fig. 3.20.1 Skin structures and infection.

Bacterial skin infections

Folliculitis is an infection of the hair follicles often caused by *Staphylococcus aureus* or, if associated with contaminated hot spa pool water, by *Pseudomonas aeruginosa*. **Furuncles** (boils) consist of walled-off collections of organisms and associated inflammatory cells in follicles and sebaceous glands that eventually 'point' and discharge pus. A rare and serious complication is the development of a cluster of boils (**carbuncle**) occurring on the neck, back or thighs, often in conjunction with fever. Recurrent boils may be associated with skin carriage of *S. aureus*, in particularly in the nose and requiring treatment with antiseptics or topical antimicrobial drugs.

Impetigo is an infection caused by *S. aureus* or *Streptococcus pyogenes* and is limited to the epidermis, presenting as yellow crusting lesions, most often on the face in young children. When the dermis is infected, a red raised demarcated rash appears (**erysipelas**), often together with fever. Certain strains of *S. pyogenes* can lead to immune-mediated kidney failure (glomerulonephritis) following infection.

'Scalded skin syndrome' is an acute infection of babies and young children caused by a staphylococcal toxin and affecting the epidermis, leading to large areas of skin loss.

Wound infections may develop after a traumatic or surgical wound gets infected with bacteria (e.g. *S. aureus*). The wound is typically red, swollen and hot to the touch. Necrotic tissue or foreign materials (including sutures) enhance bacterial growth and should be surgically removed (debrided). Localized 'walled-off' infection leads to the formation of an abscess, which will need drainage.

Some organisms release gas (e.g. *Clostridium* spp.) into the tissue (**gas gangrene**), which may be detected clinically as crepitus or seen in soft tissue radiographs. This typically follows trauma, ischaemia or contaminated surgery such as lower-limb amputation.

Wound infections or even minor skin abrasions may be complicated by the spreading of bacteria (*S. aureus, S. pyogenes*) beneath the dermis and involving subcutaneous fat (**cellulitis**). This severe condition may occur at any site but commonly involves the legs and presents with a demarcated red lesion, often with blisters. The patient is usually systemically unwell (febrile and tachycardic). Non-vitalized tissue leads to necrosis (dead tissue) and gangrene. Widespread necrosis of deeper tissues is seen in the life-threatening **necrotizing fasciitis** caused by toxin-producing 'flesh-eating bugs' (e.g. *S. pyogenes*).

Synergistic gangrene is a polymicrobial infection (multiple different bacteria) that leads to necrosis of the groin and genital

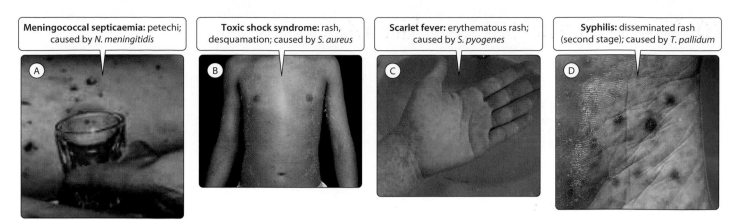

Fig. 3.20.2 Systemic bacterial infections with skin features. A. Meningococcal septicaemia *(Neisseria meningitidis)* with petechi. B. Toxic shock syndrome *(Staphylococcus aureus)* with rash and desquamation. C. Scarlet fever *(Streptococcus pyogenes)* with an erythematous rash. D. Syphilis *(Trepenoma pallidum)* with a disseminated rash in second stage (Reproduced with permission from Spicer W J 2008 Clinical microbiology and infectious diseases, 2edn, Churchill Livingstone, Edinburgh).

soft tissue. Necrotizing or gangrenous conditions require antibiotics and extensive debridement to avoid a fatal outcome.

Bites from humans (and 'clenched fist injuries'), dogs, cats, other pets and wild animals may lead to local or systemic bacterial infections. Typical causative organisms are staphylococci, streptococci and anaerobes. Infections with *Pasteurella multocida* is common following dog and cat bites.

Mycobacterial infections of the skin in primary infection with *M. tuberculosis* (lupus vulgaris) is rare, whereas *M. leprae* classically causes red anaesthetic lesions on the face, body and limbs in tuberculoid leprosy (Ch. 15). Other skin infections may be caused by atypical mycobacteria, notably the 'fish-tank' or 'swimming pool' granuloma (*M. marinum*) or the necrotizing tropical Buruli ulcer (*M. ulcerans*).

Fungal skin infections

Candidal infection of the skin is common and often associated with moist sites where skin folds rub together (**intertrigo**, e.g. nappy rash). *Candida* spp. can also infect the nail bed (**paronychia**).

'Ringworm' (**tinea**) is a localized infection of the keratinous epithelium caused by dermatophytes. These arise from human, animal or soil sources and infect skin or hair to produce circular scaly lesions. Depending on the site of infection, the infections are referred to as tinea captitis (scalp), tinea corporis (body trunk), tinea cruris (groin) or tinea pedis (feet; athlete's foot). These infections can be caused by different dermatophyte species: *Trichophyton*, *Microsporon*, *Epidermophyton* spp. or the

yeast *Malassezia furfur*, the last causing a skin infection known as **pityriasis versicolor**.

Invasive fungal infections that are prevalent in the tropics and subtropics may also present as skin lesions (e.g. *Histoplasma capsulare*).

Investigations and treatment

For bacterial infections, pus swabs or preferably infected tissue should be sent for investigation. In systemic (febrile) illness, blood cultures are essential. Adequate treatment requires drainage of pus and debridement of necrotic tissue. A Gram stain result may aid initial empirical antibiotic therapy. Most staphylococcal infections can be treated with flucloxacillin whereas *S. pyogenes* infections should respond to penicillin. Both conditions may be treated with macrolides in penicillin-allergic patients. Cefuroxime, metronidazole and gentamicin might be used where polymicrobial infections are suspected.

Animal or humans bites must be carefully explored, and antibiotic prophylaxis (e.g. co-amoxiclav) may be given.

Dermatophyte infections are diagnosed by microscopy, demonstrating fungal elements in skin scrapings, hair or nail clipping and after several weeks of culture. Many superficial fungal infections respond to topical agents such as azoles (clotrimazole, miconazole), terbinafine or selenium sulphide (for pityriasis versicolor). Severe infections or involvement of hair and nails may require oral antifungal drugs (e.g. itraconazole, terbinafine, griseofulvin). Yeasts (e.g. *Candida* spp.) are easily cultured and usually respond to topical or systemic azoles.

21. Gastrointestinal infections

Questions
- What are common causes of gastrointestinal infection?
- What are the clinical features and management of colitis?
- What are the sources of food poisoning in the UK?

Epidemiology

Gastrointestinal tract infections are among the most commonly reported diseases worldwide, causing considerable morbidity and mortality. Although most prevalent in countries where sanitation and drinking water quality are poor, intestinal infections are common in the UK (Fig. 3.21.1). All parts of the gastrointestinal tract are susceptible to infection by a variety of microorganisms and, with the exception of certain nematodes that penetrate the skin, infection arises from ingestion:

- directly from an infected human or animal by hand to mouth (faecal–oral)
- indirectly from contaminated food or water
- by consumption of food in which microbes have multiplied (food poisoning).

Although the gastrointestinal tract is vulnerable to infection, it is also well defended. The acidity of the stomach fluids (pH 2.0) is a barrier to most microbes and stops entry of pathogens into the intestinal tract. The small and large intestines are rich in commensal bacterial flora, which prevent pathogen colonization (the colon may contain 10^{12} bacteria/g faeces). Secretory IgA and lymphoid tissue (Peyer's patches) in the small intestine also provide immune protection.

Clinical features and management

Intestinal infections are diagnosed by the detection of organisms in faecal specimens using electron microscopy, immunoassay or gene detection for viruses, culture and biochemical identification of bacteria, and microscopy and immunoassays for protozoa and helminths.

Gastritis

Gastritis and peptic ulcers are associated with infections by *Helicobacter pylori*, which can colonize the stomach despite the acidic environment because it produces buffering ammonia by urease activity. Combination therapy with amoxicillin, clarithromycin and a proton pump inhibitor usually clears the infection within 1 week.

Gastroenteritis

Gastroenteritis refers to a collection of symptoms that includes nausea, vomiting, diarrhoea and abdominal discomfort. Symptoms vary with the type of organism and health of the person. The young, old or immunosuppressed are particularly susceptible to severe illness, which may be life threatening. Norovirus (winter vomiting disease) and rotavirus are transmitted by projectile vomiting and diarrhoea. Rotavirus affects mainly infants, whereas norovirus spreads in closed communities (hospital wards, cruise ships). Common causes are summarized in Fig. 3.21.2. Chapter 32 discusses tropical causes.

Bacterial infections are generally slow in onset, producing diarrhoea without vomiting that may last for a week or more. In contrast, viral infections and toxin-mediated food poisoning have a short incubation period and often produce both diarrhoea and vomiting, which resolves within a day or two. Gastroenteritis is usually a self-limiting infection and does not require antibiotic treatment. However *Salmonella typhi* and *paratyphi* invade the local lymph nodes and cause a bacteraemia (typhoid fever), which necessitate therapy with ciprofloxacin or ceftriaxone.

Colitis

Colitis is characterized by abdominal cramps (tenesmus) and haemorrhagic diarrhoea (dysentery). Typical pathogens are *Shigella* sp. and verotoxin-producing *Escherichia coli* (VTEC). *Clostridium difficile* can be part of the normal gut flora; however, it can overgrow in the elderly in the presence of antibiotics to which it is resistant (e.g. cephalosporins, quinolones and

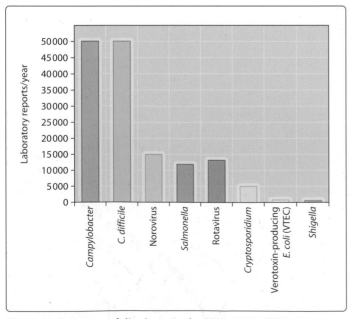

Fig. 3.21.1 Causes of diarrhoea in the UK in 2005. ETEC, enterotoxic *Escherichia coli*; VTEC, verotoxin-producing *E. coli*.

macrolides). *C. difficile* produces cytotoxins (toxin A and B) that damage the epithelial cells and induce pseudomembraneous colitis, which may present as toxic megacolon. Severe colitis requires antibiotic treatment. *C. difficile* remains sensitive to vancomycin and metronidazole, whereas *Campylobacter* and *Shigella* spp. have developed resistance to quinolones. VTEC, of which the majority in the UK is serotype O157, produces a verotoxin that not only causes colitis but also can attach to the receptors of the renal tubuli, causing haemolytic uraemic syndrome, particularly in children and the elderly.

Sources of food poisoning

Food is a common means by which pathogens can infect the gastrointestinal tract, usually as a result of contamination by an infected person during preparation. Alternatively, the organisms may be part of an animal's normal flora and contaminate the food during slaughtering and processing. However, in true food poisoning, bacteria actively multiply in the food. This does not necessarily result in spoiling of the food, which appears fit for consumption and hence increases the challenge dose and likelihood of infection:

- undercooked chicken: transmits campylobacter; incubation time 2–11 days
- raw beef or food contamination with cow dung: transmits VTEC; incubation time 1–5 days
- raw egg and its products: transmit salmonella (non-typhi); incubation time 1–3 days.

Enterotoxins can be only detected in leftover food, not in faeces.

Clinical features

Symptoms typically include both diarrhoea and vomiting and result either directly from the presence of live bacteria or from toxins produced in the food during growth. **Botulism** manifests mainly as neurological disease and less with gastrointestinal symptoms. A diagnostic algorithm based on the clinical symptoms is shown in Fig. 3.21.3.

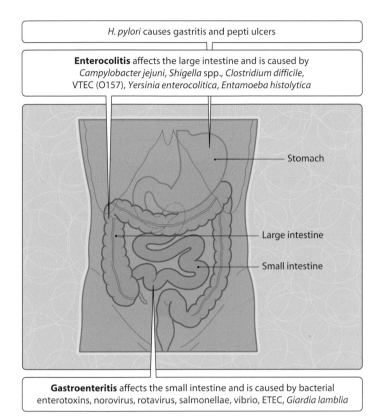

H. pylori causes gastritis and pepti ulcers

Enterocolitis affects the large intestine and is caused by *Campylobacter jejuni*, *Shigella* spp., *Clostridium difficile*, VTEC (O157), *Yersinia enterocolitica*, *Entamoeba histolytica*

Stomach

Large intestine

Small intestine

Gastroenteritis affects the small intestine and is caused by bacterial enterotoxins, norovirus, rotavirus, salmonellae, vibrio, ETEC, *Giardia lamblia*

Fig. 3.21.2 Gastrointestinal infections and their aetiology.

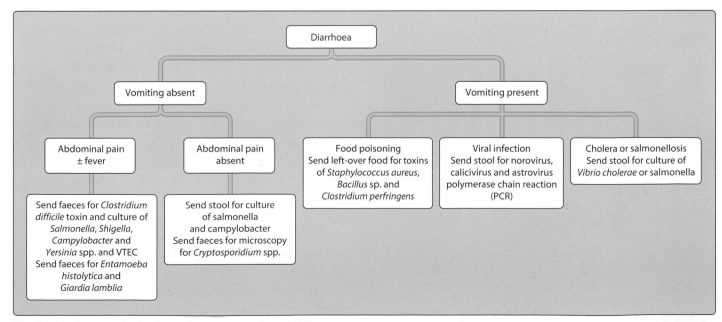

Fig. 3.21.3 Diagnostic algorithm for gastrointestinal infections.

22. Liver and pancreatic infections

Questions
- What are the clinical features of hepatitis?
- How is the laboratory diagnosis of viral hepatitis made?
- What are the causes of hepatobiliary infection?

Infection of the liver and pancreas occurs via the bloodstream, rarely from the gastrointestinal tract, even when the route of acquisition is faecal–oral. Biliary tract infection and peritonitis are, conversely, caused by locally spread infection.

Hepatitis

The classic clinical triad of jaundice, dark urine and pale stools (Fig. 3. 22.1) accompanying fever is often missing, particularly in children, who are more often asymptomatic. The vast majority of cases have a viral aetiology, with hepatitis A, B and C being the commonest causes.

Hepatitis A is spread by the faecal–oral route, has a prodrome of approximately 2–4 weeks and patients usually recover completely, although approximately 1% develop fulminant disease, which can lead to early death.

Hepatitis B is spread sexually and via contaminated blood and serous fluid. It has an incubation period of 1–3 months before patients exhibit fatigue and other classic symptoms of hepatitis. Immune-complex disease may occur, with an urticarial rash, arthritis and glomerulonephritis. Approximately 10% of patients become chronic carriers, with subsequent chronic hepatitis, cirrhosis and possibly hepatocellular carcinoma. Higher prevalence occurs in Southeast Asia.

Hepatitis C is also blood borne and has an incubation period of 2–4 months. Approximately 90% become carriers with the same long-term damage that occurs with hepatitis B.

Hepatitis D is a defective virus that only causes infection in the presence of another virus, usually hepatitis B or herpes simplex. It can recur.

Hepatitis E is spread by the faecal–oral route and is associated with water-borne epidemics. It has an incubation period of 6–8 weeks and has a high (20%) mortality in pregnant women if acquired in the third trimester, caused by the development of disseminated intravascular coagulation.

Less common causes of viral hepatitis include cytomegalovirus, Epstein–Barr virus, herpes simplex, rubella and yellow fever. There are usually other features in addition with these diseases.

Leptospira interrogans is a spirochaete that enters through the skin and causes leptospirosis, also known as Weil's disease. Sewerage workers classically get the infection from coming into contact with infected rat urine. It can also spread through the faecal–oral route and may be complicated by aseptic meningitis and haemorrhage.

Entamoeba histolytica and parasitic infections are common causes of hepatitis in tropical climates.

Approximately 10% of cases of hepatitis do not have an identifiable cause, and new viruses such as hepatitis G and TT virus have been discovered by modern molecular methods in some cases. Their aetiological role has, however, yet to be defined.

Diagnosis and management

Diagnosis of viral (and leptospiral) infection is serological, by detection of either antigen or specific antibody. The detection of hepatitis B surface antigen (HBsAg) confirms the diagnosis of hepatitis B virus, and the presence of hepatitis B 'e' antigen (HBeAg) indicates a high infectious risk (Fig. 3.22.2). Other markers are determined in specific cases. Jaundice in carriers, in whom HBsAg persists for 6 months or more, is most likely to have another cause, which should be sought. Hepatitis A virus infection is diagnosed by specific IgM. Serological assays for the diagnosis of hepatitis C do not offer early diagnosis, as they are based on the detection of specific IgG, which may take several weeks to develop; diagnosis is, therefore, retrospective unless an earlier method such as gene amplification in the polymerase chain reaction is used.

Management of acute viral hepatitis is supportive, with bed rest at the peak of liver inflammation. Chronic hepatitis therapy is evolving, with drugs such as interferon, immunomodulators and ribavirin being used with moderate success in delaying

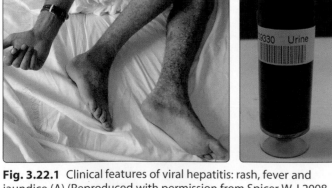

Fig. 3.22.1 Clinical features of viral hepatitis: rash, fever and jaundice (A) (Reproduced with permission from Spicer W J 2008 Clinical microbiology and infectious diseases, 2edn, Churchill Livingstone, Edinburgh) and dark urine (B).

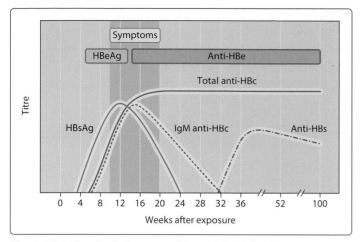

Fig. 3.22.2 Serological course of hepatitis B infection. HBsAg, hepatitis B surface antigen; HBeAg, hepatitis B early antigen; HBc, hepatitis B core antigen.

progression of liver disease, although viral eradication is not achieved. Prevention of infection involves public health measures and vaccination for hepatitis A and hepatitis B. Travellers from the UK to areas of higher prevalence (outside northern and western Europe and North America) should consider vaccination for hepatitis A. Although universal vaccination for hepatitis B is being introduced in several countries, in the UK it is targeted at higher-risk groups, such as medical, nursing and laboratory staff; homosexual men; and residents of mental institutions. Passive immunization is available for susceptible individuals in the event of contacts with either hepatitis A or hepatitis B.

Leptospirosis is treated with pencillin, and antiparasitic drugs are used in those caused by such organisms.

Liver abscess

Liver abscesses may be primary infections or secondary to haematogenous spread from another site. Usually bacterial, with mixed anaerobic and aerobic flora (including Enterobacteriaceae and *Streptococcus milleri* group), abscesses consist of pus that has been walled off by a fibrinous layer; this can be detected by imaging. Single lesions are often asymptomatic unless very large. Broad-spectrum antibiotics are used to treat the condition, but surgical drainage may also be required.

Biliary tract infection

Biliary tract infection can occur secondary to obstruction, by either gallstones or malignancy. Ascending cholangitis, liver abscess and septicaemia may be sequelae. Diagnosis is clinical, with imaging used as a confirmatory test. Treatment consists of removal of the obstruction and broad-spectrum antibiotics.

Peritonitis

Contamination of the sterile peritoneal cavity occurs through breach of the bowel or urogenital wall. This may be iatrogenic, such as occurs in surgery, or through diseases such as inflammatory bowel disease, appendicitis and malignancy. Occasionally tuberculosis or actinomycosis of the genital tract may have been the initial site of infection. Genital chlamydia and gonococcal infections can also ascend to cause perihepatitis (so-called **FitzHugh–Curtis syndrome**). Clinical diagnosis is confirmed operatively, or through laparoscopy, with pus and/or adhesions visible between the peritoneal layers. Treatment with broad-spectrum antibiotics may be required as infections arising from the gut are polymicrobial.

Pancreatitis

Pancreatitis can be caused by a number of viruses: mumps, enteroviruses; cytomegalovirus, Epstein–Barr virus. Mumps is the commonest. Diabetes mellitus is associated with preceding enterovirus infection. Bacteria can cause pancreatitis, with mixed flora, if there is obstruction at the ampulla of Vater, usually by malignancy.

23. Infections of the heart

Questions
- Who is at risk of endocarditis?
- What are the clinical signs of endocarditis?
- What is the clinical management?

Endocarditis

Epidemiology

The incidence of bacterial endocarditis increases from 3/100 000 of the population to 10/100 000 for people aged over 65 years. Valvular abnormalities, particularly those that damage the endothelial surface by high-velocity jets (audible as a murmur), predispose to a fibrin–platelet deposit. Patients who had endocarditis previously or have prosthetic heart valves are also at risk. An intermittent bacteraemia (e.g. caused by injury or inflammation of the mucosal surfaces in the mouth, gastrointestinal or genitourinary tract) seeds the preformed thrombus, which enlarges to a **vegetation**. *Streptococcus viridans*, enterococci, *Staphylococcus aureus* and the so-called HACEK group (oral fastidious Gram-negative rods) have particular affinity for fibrinonectin in the thrombus. Patients in high-risk group, (prosthetic heart valves, congenital heart disease and previous endocarditis) should receive antibiotic prophylaxis on induction for surgery that is potentially contaminated and dirty. Usually amoxicillin and gentamicin is given.

Clinical features

Patients with infective endocarditis present with non-specific symptoms such as fever, night sweats, arthralgias and usually a murmur. Infected valvular vegetations result in local tissue destruction, embolic events and formation of immune complexes. Valve destruction may present as new regurgitation or conduction block. Embolic events lead to the characteristic splinter haemorrhages (Fig. 3.23.1), Janeway lesions and cerebral and pulmonary infarcts. Immunological phenomena comprise painful Osler nodes on fingers, arthritis and glomerulonephritis.

Diagnosis

Echocardiography (Fig. 3.23.2) is the mainstay of diagnosis. Transthoracic echocardiography (TTE) is less sensitive (70%) than transoesophageal echocardiography (TOE), but more readily availabe in hospitals. Patients with abnormal native valves, prosthetic valves or calcification require TOE for imaging of vegetation or abscesses. Three to six blood cultures should be collected from different venepuncture sites within 24 h (spaced at least 1 h apart) before commencing antibiotic therapy. For the

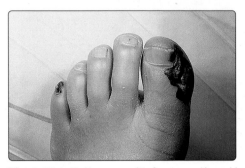

Fig. 3.23.1 Splinters and infarcts produced by embolization in infective endocarditis. (Reproduced with permission from Spicer W J 2008 Clinical microbiology and infectious diseases, 2edn, Churchill Livingstone, Edinburgh.)

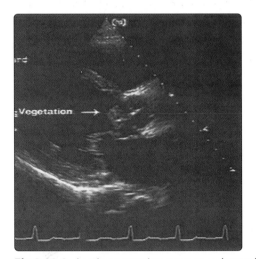

Fig 3.23.2 Aortic vegetation seen on echocardiography.

diagnosis of microorganisms that usually do not grow in blood cultures (*Coxiella burnetii*, *Bartonella* spp. and *Chlamydophila psitacii*), serological investigations should be performed. As symptoms are non-specific (Fig. 3.23.3), modified Dukes criteria have been developed to improve the diagnosis by weighting clinical symptoms. Division is made into whether a native or prosthetic valve is involved and the latter by time of onset: early (within 2 months of surgery) or late.

Management

The importance of obtaining an isolate is that detailed susceptibility studies are significant in optimizing antimicrobial treatment. The **minimum inhibitory concentration** (MIC) of antibacterial drugs should be determined to ensure appropriate doses and duration of therapy. In most cases, combination therapy is employed to provide enhanced activity; for example the addition of gentamicin to benzylpenicillin improves bactericidal activity against many streptococci and enterococci.

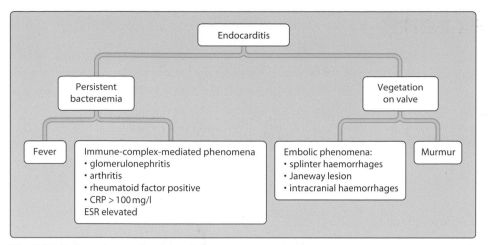

Fig. 3.23.3 Symptoms of endocarditis.

High-dose regimens for 4–6 weeks are required for successful therapy, and clinicians should liaise closely with microbiologists to select and monitor therapy. Antibiotic levels (e.g. gentamicin, vancomycin) need monitoring closely, and serial measurements of C-reactive protein, white cell count and temperature are helpful in assessing response. Despite appropriate antimicrobial therapy, the attributable mortality remains 20%. Where extensive valvular damage or recurrent embolic events have occurred (and in most cases of prosthetic disease), valve replacement may be required in addition to antimicrobial therapy

Myocarditis and pericarditis

Infection of the heart muscle or pericardium is often viral (enterovirus, influenza, rubella, Epstein–Barr virus, cytomegalovirus) in origin, although pericarditis may develop in severe bacterial infection with *Staphylococcus aureus*, pneumococci, group A streptococci, Q-fever, *Mycoplasma pneumoniae* and *Mycobacterium tuberculosis*. Typical symptoms include a flu-like illness and localized pain. Myocarditis may cause arrhythmia and, in severe cases, heart failure. In pericarditis, a pericardial rub may be heard and, in severe cases, typically caused by pyogenic bacteria, effusion may be demonstrated by chest radiography or echocardiography. Respiratory swabs and stool samples should be cultured for viruses, and blood and pericardial fluid (where available) cultured for bacteria. Viral infections are usually self-limiting, but bacterial pericarditis requires pericardial drainage and prompt antibiotic treatment.

CASE STUDY: Endocarditis

A 70-year-old man presented with a facial palsy to the emergency department. He had been suffering from night sweats for 4 weeks, had swollen wrists and ankles and a painful non-blanching macula on his right palm. On examination, he had a right-sided facial palsy, no lymphadenopathy and a few splinters under the fingernails of his right thumb and left digit finger. He had hepatosplenomegaly and a systolic murmur. His temperature was 38°C, C-reactive protein 160 mg/l, white blood cell count 8.4×10^9/l and platelets 15×10^9/l. Rheumatoid factor was positive; however antineutrophil cytoplasmic antibodies (ANCA) and antinuclear factor (ANA) were negative. Two blood cultures collected at admission grew *Streptococcus bovis,* which was sensitive to penicillin and ceftriaxone. Echocardiogram revealed a large vegetation on the aortic valve. Ultrasound of the abdomen confirmed hepatosplenomegaly and found a hypodense lesion in the spleen, which was suggestive of an infarct. Computed tomography of the brain showed a ring-enhancing lesion consistent with a brain abscess.

A diagnosis was made of infective endocarditis of the aortic valve caused by *S. bovis* and complicated by septic emboli in spleen and brain. The lesion in the palm was a Janeway lesion. The arthritis and the positive rheumatoid factor were most likely manifestations of circulating IgM antibodies to *S. bovis.* The patient was treated with intravenous benzylpenicillin and low-dose gentamicin to sterilize the vegetation on the valve, which requires 4–6 weeks of intravenous therapy. As *S. bovis* bacteraemia is associated with colon carcinoma, he underwent colonoscopy, which did not reveal any tumour.

Two weeks after starting the intravenous therapy, he had a second embolic event in his brain and was referred to a cardiothoracic unit for aortic valve replacement. Large vegetations of more than 1 cm in diameter tend to cause septic emboli and often require valve replacement. He recovered fully after this procedure in a rehabilitation hospital.

24. Urinary tract infections

Questions
- Who is at risk of a urinary tract infection?
- How is uncomplicated urinary tract infection defined?
- How is the diagnosis of a urinary tract infection made?
- Which empirical antibiotic treatment is effective?

Urinary tract infections (UTI) are more common at certain ages (Fig. 3.24.1). While many infections are mild, renal infections may lead to long-term kidney damage, and the urinary tract is a common source of life-threatening Gram-negative bacteraemia. Risk factors for UTI in infants and children are anatomical and functional anomalies (e.g. ureteric reflux, strictures, neurogenic bladder). Women have a shorter urethra than men and so are more prone to bladder infection, particularly after intercourse. Any obstruction to urine flow can predispose to infection. In pregnancy, the ureter is dilated and can be obstructed by the gravid uterus. In elderly men, prostate enlargement obstructs the urethra and in elderly women a cystocele can lead to residual urine volumes in the bladder. Catheterization introduces exogenous flora, which in hospital are often multiresistant. Figure 3.24.2 shows the likely infecting species in the hospital setting and in the community.

Clinical features
Several clinical syndromes are recognized (Fig. 3.24.3). If women present with dysuria, frequency and suprapubic pain, the probability of uncomplicated UTI is high. If fewer symptoms are present, the **urethral syndrome** is possible, which is a lower UTI without 'significant bacteriuria'. The aetiology of this condition is controversial but chlamydial infections may play a role.

Asymptomatic bacteriuria (bacteriuria $> 10^5$ colony-forming units (CFU)/ml in the absence of pyuria) occurs in approximately 5% of women and is important in pregnancy, where 20–30% will develop acute pyelonephritis if untreated. Bacteriuria in pregnancy is also associated with premature birth, low birthweight and increased perinatal mortality. It is, therefore, important that all women have their urine cultured early in pregnancy.

Diagnosis
Urine specimens need to be collected with care to minimize contamination with perineal organisms. The first portion of voided urine is discarded and a **midstream urine** (MSU) specimen collected. Specimens from catheterized patients should be collected by needle aspiration from the catheter tubing. In children, specimens may be collected in adhesive bags, but suprapubic aspiration may be required to avoid contamination. Where there may be a delay in examination, specimens should be refrigerated or collected in containers with boric acid to prevent bacterial multiplication in transit. **Dipstick tests** are available for the detection of blood, leukocyte esterase (indicating white blood cells) and nitrite (indicating the presence of nitrate-reducing bacteria). The absence of nitrite and/or leukoesterase excludes cystitis in women (Fig. 3.24.4). For the diagnosis of UTI in men, children and in pregnancy, significant bacteriuria in culture should be demonstrated.

Microscopy for white and red blood cells may be helpful in the interpretation of culture results, but their presence does not necessarily indicate urinary tract infection. Squamous epithelial cells usually indicate contamination of the specimen. The normal urinary tract is sterile, but urine may be contaminated with organisms from the distal urethra during voiding.

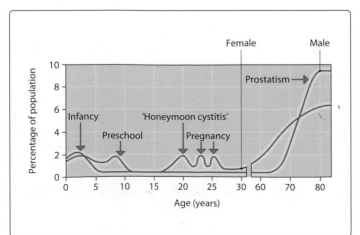

Fig. 3.24.1 Prevalence of urinary tract infection by age.

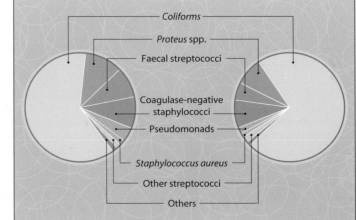

Fig. 3.24.2 Urine isolates in hospital (left) and general practice (right).

Kass defined the term **significant bacteriuria** as > 10⁵ CFU/ml for a single organism. This figure was derived from studies in women and was found to distinguish pyelonephritis from contamination. However, despite regular usage since, this figure has not been validated for other urinary infections or those in men or children. In patients with symptomatic infections, counts may be as low as 10² CFU/ml.

Quantitative culture is followed by susceptibility testing of significant isolates. The interpretation of culture results depends on clinical details (symptoms, previous antibiotics), quality of specimen, delay in culture and species isolated. Repeat specimens are required for asymptomatic bacteriuria. **Sterile pyuria**—white blood cells in the urine in the absence of bacterial growth—may be caused by prior antibiotics, urethritis (chlamydia or gonococci), vaginal infections or urinary tuberculosis. Where tuberculosis is considered, three early morning urine specimens should be collected for culture when the urine is most concentrated. All patients with long-term catheters have bacteriuria and frequently pyuria as a result of the bladder irritation by the foreign body. The diagnosis in patients with a catheter relies more on clinical symptoms (e.g. fever and/or confusion).

Treatment

Uncomplicated cystitis should be treated with a short (typically 3 days) course of an oral antibacterial agent such as trimethoprim or nitrofurantoin, depending on local resistance rates. Post-treatment follow-up cultures are particularly important in children and pregnant women. For patients with **complicated infections**, antibiotics such as quinolones or gentamicin are often indicated, depending on antibiotic susceptibility. **Pyelonephritis** requires treatment, initially systemic, for a total of 10–14 days, or with ciprofloxacin for 7 days. **Asymptomatic bacteriuria** in pregnancy should be treated with cephalosporins or nitrofurantoin for 7 days. Antimicrobial treatment is usually only recommended in patients with indwelling catheters and systemic features of infection. The catheter should be removed whenever possible. In some patients, a prophylactic dose of an antibacterial agent given at night may reduce the incidence of **recurrent cystitis**.

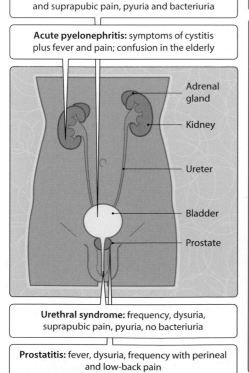

Fig. 3.24.3 Clinical syndromes of urinary tract infection.

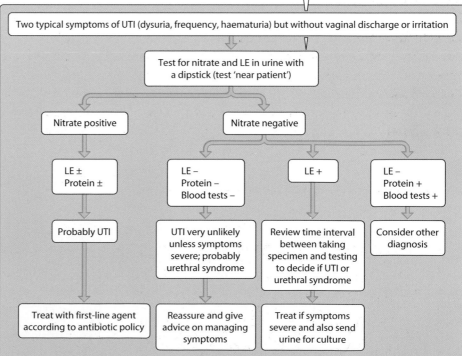

Fig. 3.24.4 Diagnostic and treatment algorithm for uncomplicated urinary tract infection (UTI) in women.

25. Genital tract infections

Questions
- Which genital tract infections are common?
- Which are the infectious agents of urethritis?
- Which are the infectious agents of genital ulcers?

Host susceptibility and epidemiology

Genital tract infections includes a number of sexually transmitted diseases (STDs), as well as some infections that do not require sexual activity for transmission. The STDs where the main symptoms occur outside the genital tract (e.g. HIV and hepatitis B) are considered elsewhere. In the male, with the exception of the distal 2–3 cm, the normal urethra is sterile, protected by mucus, prostatic secretions and periodic flushing with urine. The commensal flora of the vagina offers some protective effect, as does the mucus within the cervix and uterine cell turnover through menstruation. STDs require intimate contact for transmission. Contact tracing is undertaken following diagnosis to reduce transmission within the community; GPs will often refer patients to the local genitourinary clinic where all the facilities are available. Chlamydial and human papillomavirus infections are highly endemic among 16–24 year olds (Fig. 3.25.1).

The clinical syndromes

There are few clinical presentations: skin infections present in both sexes in the same way, whereas other genital infections manifest in different organs depending on gender (Fig. 3.25.2). Table 3.25.1 gives the methods of diagnosis and treatments.

Skin infections

Herpes simplex infection is a relapsing condition that produces multiple painful ulcers on the genital skin and mucous membranes following a variable prodrome of tingling. Human papillomavirus infection is generally a self-limiting condition marked by non-painful warts or dry scaling lesions on the genital skin; although it is less obvious, mucosal surfaces may also be infected with certain types of virus, bringing an increased risk of carcinoma, particularly of the cervix.

Syphilis is a multisystem disorder, now rare, caused by the spirochaete *Treponema pallidum*. Three ulcerative conditions with regional lymphadenopathy are more common in the tropics: chancroid (*Haemophilus ducreyi*), granuloma inguinale (*Klebsiella granulomatis*) and lymphogranuloma venereum (*Chlamydia trachomatis* serotypes L1–L3).

Infection in the male

Urethritis in males is usually symptomatic, with discharge and dysuria. *C. trachomatis* serotypes D–K are the most common cause, although more severe symptoms suggest infection with *Neisseria gonorrhoeae*. Mixed infections are possible. Urethritis may progress to involve the prostate or epididymis, which may be more difficult to treat. Reiter's syndrome (urethritis, iritis and arthritis) is an unpleasant relapsing condition that may follow an episode of urethritis, particularly in *HLA-B27* carriers.

Table 3.25.1 GENITAL TRACT INFECTIONS

Infection	Cause	Diagnosis	Treatment
Genital warts	Human papilloma virus (HPV)	Clinical, PCR	Chemical or surgical removal, imiquimod
Genital herpes	Herpes simplex virus type 2	Viral culture, PCR	Aciclovir
Cervicitis/ urethritis	*N. gonorrhoeae*, *C. trachomatis* serotypes D–K	PCR for chlamydia, microscopy and culture for *N. gonorrhoeae*	*C. trachomatis*: doxycycline or azithromycin *N. gonorrhoeae*: ceftriaxone
Syphilitic chancre	*T. pallidum*	Dark field microscopy, serology	Penicillin
Chancroid	*H. ducreyi*	Culture, PCR	Azithromycin
Lympho-granuloma venereum	*C. trachomatis* serotypes L1–L3	Serology	Doxycycline
Granuloma inguinale	*K. granulomatis*	Microscopy	Azithromycin

PCR, polymerase chain reaction.

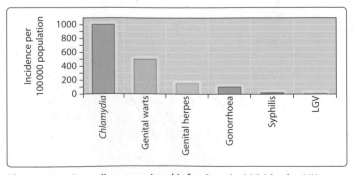

Fig. 3.25.1 Sexually transmitted infections in 2006 in the UK among 16–24 year olds. LVG, lymphogranuloma venereum.

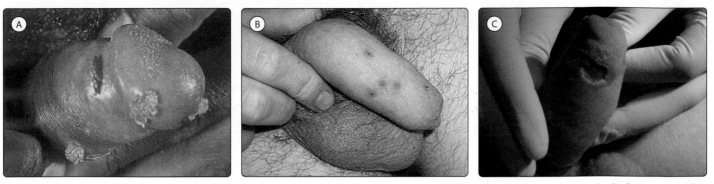

Fig. 3.25.2 A. Genital warts (human papilloma virus) found around the anus, vagina, vulva or cervix and on the penis shaft. B. Gential herpes (herpes simplex type 2). C. Syphilitic chancre (*T. pallidum*). (courtesy of Dr R. Nadarajan, Frimley park Hospital, Frimley, UK.)

Proctitis is most common amongst male homosexuals, with rectal pain, bleeding and discharge. Recently, rectal lymphogranuloma venereum has occurred among homosexuals in European.

Infection in the female

Silent infections are common in women. *N. gonorrhoeae* may cause infection of Bartholin's glands at the vaginal introitus, although other bacteria can also be responsible. **Vaginal discharge** is a common reason for medical consultation, and an accurate diagnosis may be obtained from a vaginal swab (Table 3.25.2). Candidiasis is common and more likely with the oral contraceptives, pregnancy, diabetes and following the use of antibiotics. Similarly, **anaerobic** or **bacterial vaginosis** is caused by a disturbance in the normal vaginal flora, often following the use of broad-spectrum antibiotics. If the problem is seen to arise from the cervical os and not the vagina, samples of the discharge should be sent for more-detailed analysis. The causes of **cervicitis** are all sexually transmitted, with chlamydia being the most common. While infection may often be asymptomatic, it is still a reservoir for spread to others and ascending infection.

Pelvic inflammatory disease may present as an acute peritonitis, as chronic pelvic pain and dyspareunia or be clinically silent. There is a significant risk of damage to the Fallopian tubes, leading to an increased incidence of ectopic pregnancy and infertility. Treatment often involves the 'blind' use of antibiotic cover, including for chlamydial infection (e.g. ofloxacin and metronidazole) as a microbiological diagnosis is unlikely without laparoscopy.

Table 3.25.2 VAGINAL DISCHARGE

Symptom	Infectious agent	Diagnosis	Treatment
White creamy discharge, pruritus	*Candida albicans*	Microscopy, culture	Topical clotrimazole, oral fluconazole
Foul-smelling discharge	Bacterial vaginosis (*Gardnerella* and anaerobes)	Microscopy	Metronidazole
Frothy copious discharge	*Trichomonas vaginalis*	Microscopy, culture	Metronidazole

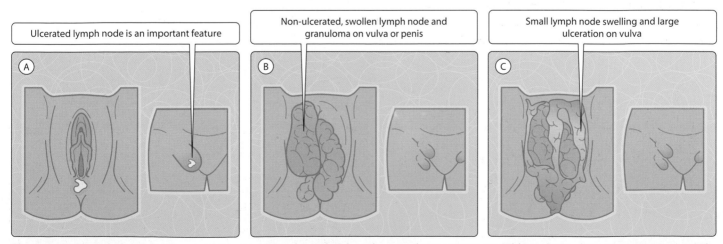

| Ulcerated lymph node is an important feature | Non-ulcerated, swollen lymph node and granuloma on vulva or penis | Small lymph node swelling and large ulceration on vulva |

Fig. 3.25.3 Genital ulcers. A. Chancroid (*Haemophilus ducreyi*); B. lymphogranuloma venereum (*Chlamydia trachomatis* serotypes L1–L3); C. granuloma inguinale (donovaniosis; *Klebsiella granulomatis*).

26. Obstetric and neonatal infections

Questions
- Which infections are transmitted vertically to the fetus?
- How can intrauterine infections be diagnosed?
- How can perinatal infections be prevented?

Both the pregnant woman and the newborn infant are to some extent immunocompromised. Most infections in pregnancy are not more common (an exception is urinary tract infection) but are more likely to be severe (particularly chickenpox, viral hepatitis and malaria). Primary infection in the mother induces IgM antibodies but these do not pass through the placenta to the fetus. Intrauterine infection may result in fetal death and spontaneous abortion or **congenital** infection and associated malformations. The baby may also acquire infection around the time of birth (perinatal infection) or after birth (postnatal infection) (Fig. 3.26.1). **Puerperal** infections are postnatal infections in the mother.

Congenital infections

Most congenital infections may also cause spontaneous abortion. TORCH is an acronym for the infections of toxoplasma, rubella, cytomegalovirus and herpes simplex. It is a useful aide mémoire but is by no means all inclusive. Acute maternal *Toxoplasma gondii* infection is usually asymptomatic; however it can cause transplacental infection of the fetus. Primary toxoplasmosis in pregnancy can result, in a minority, in congenital damage with hydrocephalus, intracranial calcifications and chorioretinitis (Fig. 3.26.2). The diagnosis can be confirmed by amniocentesis; antiparasitic therapy needs to be continued in infancy. Most infants who are infected while in the womb have no symptoms at birth but may develop symptoms later in life.

Infections causing skin rashes and carrying a risk for congenital infections if they occur in pregnancy comprise rubella virus (German measles), varicella zoster virus (VZV; chickenpox) and parvovirus. Primary maternal rubella infection in the first trimester carries a high risk of **congenital rubella syndrome** (microcephalus, cataract, deafness and heart defects) in the fetus, resulting in termination of pregnancy in many cases. Vaccination in childhood has been introduced for prevention. Primary VZV infection in the first 20 weeks of gestation can cause **congenital varicella syndrome** (eye defects, hypoplastic limb, microcephalus), but in less than 2% (Fig. 3.26.3). VZV infection around delivery can cause neonatal varicella syndrome (rash, pneumonitis) and severe maternal varicella zoster pneumonitis, which can be treated with high doses of intravenous aciclovir. Giving VZV immunoglobulins to mother or neonate within 7 to 10 days of exposure may prevent fetal and neonatal varicella zoster syndrome. Parvovirus infections during the first 20 weeks of gestation cause fetal anaemia and hydrops in less than 10%, and can be diagnosed by cordocentesis and monitoring for fetal ascites.

Maternal primary **cytomegalovirus infection** (but also reactivation) can cause deafness or retardation in the fetus, although in less than 7%. Diagnosis of congenital infection can be made by

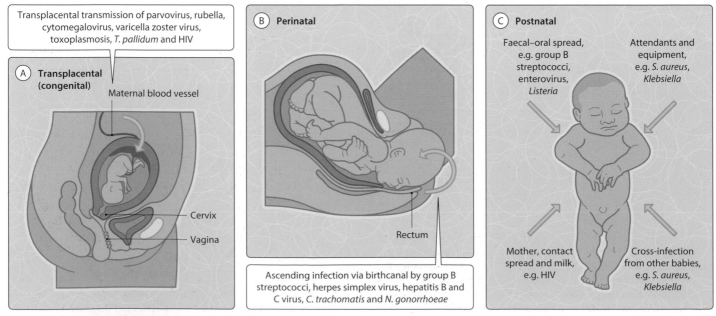

Fig. 3.26.1 Routes of fetal and neonatal infections.

the polymerase chain reaction on amniotic fluid or postnatally within 3 weeks of birth on neonatal blood or urine.

Syphilis has become rare in developed countries; however, as it is treatable with penicillin during pregnancy, it is still part of the antenatal serological screen together with HIV, hepatitis B and rubella.

Perinatal infections

Most perinatal pathogens arise from the birth canal or blood. Although blood-borne viruses can be transmitted intrauterinely, the highest risk is during delivery. **HIV** transmission can be reduced by peripartum antiretroviral therapy, elective caesarian section and avoidance of breastfeeding. Perinatal **hepatitis B** infection can be prevented by vaccination of the newborn as soon as possible after birth. Neonates with viraemic mothers require immunoglobulins against hepatitis B in addition to vaccine. The risk of vertical transmission of **hepatitis C** may be reduced by elective caesarian section; in the absence of a vaccine, the infant needs to be monitored for viraemia and treated with antiviral drugs if it develops. **Herpes simplex virus** (HSV) can be transmitted from mother to child. Lesions may be present at the time of delivery. Neonatal HSV infection can be disseminated and cause encephalitis (Fig. 3.26.4). Elective caesarian section or perinatal aciclovir therapy may prevent vertical transmission. **Group B streptococci** silently colonize the maternal genital and gastrointestinal tracts until ascending infection produces severe and disseminated disease in the baby. Such infections are more common when there has been premature rupture of membranes. Antibiotic prophylaxis is given during labour and to the baby after birth when the mothers have a history of group B streptococcal carriage or have fever during labour. Early-onset infection in the neonate (within the first week of life) usually presents as a severe septicaemia, whereas late-onset disease often presents as meningitis. Eye infection in the newborn is known as **ophthalmia neonatorum**. Eye swabs should be collected for culture of *Neisseria gonorrhoeae* and immunofluorescence or molecular techniques detect chlamydial infections. *N. gonorrhoeae* can be treated with topical antibiotics, whereas *Chlamydia trachomatis* requires systemic erythromycin.

Postnatal infections

Infection acquired after birth may be associated with cross-infection from babies, their mothers and attendant staff in nurseries and neonatal intensive care units. Staphylococcal infections are usually minor but may present as the **scalded skin syndrome**. With suspected covert bacterial infection, blood and CSF must be cultured promptly, together with swabs of superficial sites (e.g. umbilicus, ear and rectum). Urgent antibacterial treatment should then be started (e.g. penicillin and gentamicin). Scrupulous attention to **aseptic techniques** and other infection control procedures is essential in the care of neonates.

Puerperal infections

Puerperal sepsis, caused by group A streptococci, is now uncommon since the introduction of hand washing by attendants and associated procedures. Other organisms associated with puerperal infections include anaerobes and coliforms, may be introduced during instrumentation, especially septic abortions. The risk of infection is increased if products of conception are retained in the uterus. Blood cultures and high vaginal swabs should be sent and empirical antibiotic treatment started. *Staphylococcus aureus* may cause **breast abscesses** in the mother a week or so after birth.

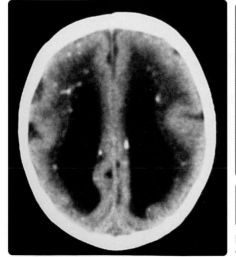

Fig. 3.26.2 Congenital toxoplasmosis is associated with hydrocephalus, intracranial calcifications and chorioretinitis. Periventricular calcifications in the brain can be seen with computed tomography.

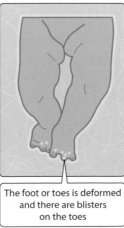

The foot or toes is deformed and there are blisters on the toes

Fig. 3.26.3 Congenital varicella syndrome: bilateral lower-limb deformities in an infant whose mother had varicella at 12 weeks of gestation.

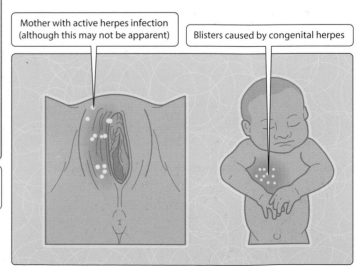

Mother with active herpes infection (although this may not be apparent)

Blisters caused by congenital herpes

Fig. 3.26.4 Disseminated neonatal herpes simplex type 2 infection: maternal infection can be transmitted perinatally and leads to a vesicular rash, with pneumonitis and encephalitis in the newborn.

27. Infections of bone, joints and muscle

Questions
- What are the sources for osteomyelitis?
- How is the diagnosis of osteomyelitis made?
- What is the difference between septic and reactive arthritis?

Osteomyelitis

Infections of bone may arise from haematogenous and exogenous sources (Fig. 3.27.1). Bacteraemias in adults, particularly with *Staphylococcus aureus* and *Brucella* sp., may seed into adjacent vertebrae with their intervertebral disc (**discitis**). In prepubertal children, the metaphysis of tibia and femur may develop small post-traumatic haematomas under the growth plate, into which occult bacteraemia may nidulate. Patients with sickle cell disease are particularly at risk of salmonella osteomyelitis. In countries where tuberculosis is endemic, mycobacteria can settle in those niduses. Exogenous entry of bacteria occurs through open fractures, deep soft tissue defects (diabetic foot ulcers, decubital ulcers) or during surgical insertion of metal plates or prostheses. Prosthetic infections occur in less than 1% of elective total joint replacements; however, they are more common after hemiarthroplasties for traumatic fractures of the neck of femur.

Clinical features and diagnosis
Haematogenous infections ususally present with fever and localized bone pain, whereas exogenous infections may have a more insidious onset, show chronic low-grade pain and may lead to mechanical

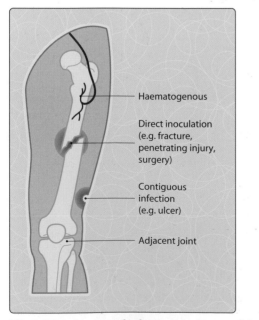

Fig. 3.27.1 Sources of infection in osteomyelitis.

Haematogenous

Direct inoculation
(e.g. fracture,
penetrating injury,
surgery)

Contiguous
infection
(e.g. ulcer)

Adjacent joint

loosening of the prosthesis or the metal plates. In over 50% of haematogenous infections, blood cultures may reveal the infectious agent. Magnetic resonance imaging can detect osteomyelitis earlier than radiography, which show bone destruction after a delay of 2–3 weeks (Fig. 3.27.2). Bone biopsy is useful for the aetiological diagnosis of the majority of exogenous infections, and joint aspirates may be contributory to the diagnosis of infected joint replacements.

Management
Osteomyelitis requires antimicrobial therapy for 4–6 weeks, which should be guided by the bacterial aetiology (Fig. 3.27.3). Flucloxacillin requires intravenous administration to achieve a therapeutic concentration in bone and can be switched to intravenous ceftriaxone once daily for outpatient therapy. A few antibiotics have good bioavailability when given orally (e.g. clindamycin, quinolones, rifampicin and doxycycline; NB fusidic acid must not be given as monotherapy). Haematogenous infections which have been treated within 2 to 3 weeks of onset can be cured by antibiotic therapy alone. However, if the onset was insidious and treatment delayed, debridement of necrotic bone tissues (sequestra) is necessary. Infected metal work or prostheses require removal, and often a two-stage revision arthroplasty is used, comprising removal of prosthesis with bone sampling for aetiological diagnosis and antibiotic spacer insertion, 6 weeks of intravenous antibiotics and then reimplantation of a new prosthesis. To prevent this costly complication, all joint replacements should be performed under antibiotic cover and in ultraclean theatres with high-efficiency particulate filtered air (HEPA).

Infective arthritis
Risk and clinical features
Most bacterial joint infections follow haematogenous spread and lead to **septic arthritis** with joint effusions, most commonly in the knee or hip. Chronic infections may develop, particularly with mycobacteria or fungi. The following clinical features may be present:
- fever (often with systemic illness)
- pain, swelling, erythema
- raised white cell count, elevated C-reactive protein.

In contrast **reactive arthritis** is sterile and caused by an immune response to an infection (postinfectious). In many cases, this follows infections (e.g. campylobacter, chlamydia, *Streptococcus pyogenes*, parvovirus, rubella virus and hepatitis B virus) and is associated with the *HLA-B27*. In viral infections (e.g. rubella), multiple joints are often involved, especially the hands, wrists, knees, ankles and elbows, and the arthropathy 'flits' from one joint to another.

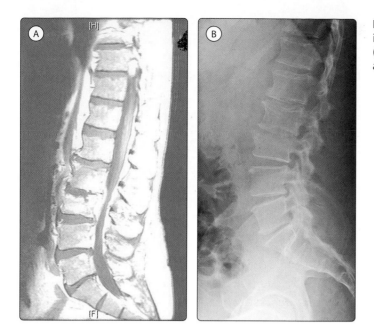

Fig. 3.27.2 Magnetic resonance image (A) shows discitis in L2/L3 and an epidural abscess. Concomitant radiograph (B) shows disc space loss between L2/L3 but not the epidural abscess.

Investigation

Radiographs show distension of the joint capsule and soft-tissue swelling; destructive changes are only seen in those who present late. These findings are not diagnostic of infection, and inflammatory conditions (e.g. rheumatoid arthritis and gout) need to be considered. Blood cultures should be taken and joint fluid aspirated. In bacterial infections, approximately 50% of aspirates show bacteria with the Gram stain and 90% are positive on culture. Patients thought to have arthritis associated with gonococci or following gastrointestinal infections should have appropriate additional specimens taken. When tuberculosis is suspected, synovial biopsies should be taken. Serology is used to determine viral infection.

Management

Acute bacterial arthritis requires 4–6 weeks of antibiotic treatment, initially for 2 weeks by the intravenous route. Open surgical drainage (joint washout) is usually necessary for large joints.

Infections of muscle

Acute bacterial cellulitis caused by group A β-haemolytic streptococci may involve underlying fascia and muscles (necrotizing fasciitis). Gangrene may follow trauma or infection with mixed organisms, including streptococci, anaerobes and coliforms. Both potentially fatal infections require prompt antibiotic therapy and full surgical debridement. **Viral myositis** produces self-limiting muscle pain and may be caused by coxsackieviruses, mumps or influenza. **Parasitic infections** include *Trypanosoma cruzi* (Chagas' disease), which may destroy cardiac muscle; *Taenia solium*, which produces calcified muscle cysts; and *Trichinella spiralis*, which causes fever and muscle pains.

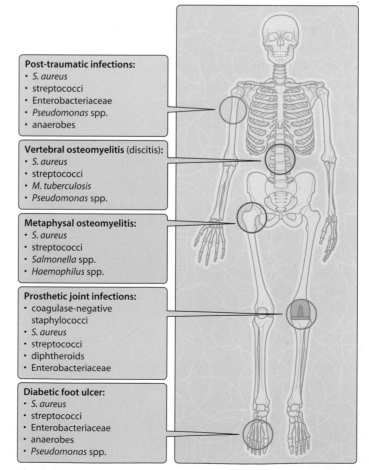

Post-traumatic infections:
• *S. aureus*
• streptococci
• Enterobacteriaceae
• *Pseudomonas* spp.
• anaerobes

Vertebral osteomyelitis (discitis):
• *S. aureus*
• streptococci
• *M. tuberculosis*
• *Pseudomonas* spp.

Metaphysal osteomyelitis:
• *S. aureus*
• streptococci
• *Salmonella* spp.
• *Haemophilus* spp.

Prosthetic joint infections:
• coagulase-negative staphylococci
• *S. aureus*
• streptococci
• diphtheroids
• Enterobacteriaceae

Diabetic foot ulcer:
• *S. aureus*
• streptococci
• Enterobacteriaceae
• anaerobes
• *Pseudomonas* spp.

Fig. 3.27.3 Aetiology of osteomyelitis.

28. Septicaemia

Questions
- What are the clinical features and possible causes of septicaemia?
- How is a blood culture taken?

Septicaemia is a clinical term describing signs of infection associated with microorganisms in the bloodstream. The term **bacteraemia** simply refers to the presence of bacteria in the blood, sometimes transiently, with or without symptoms. Septicaemia carries a high mortality and must be recognized, investigated and treated promptly.

Aetiology

There are a number of different risk factors associated with community- or hospital-acquired septicaemia. The incidence of many community-acquired infections has changed little in recent years, and typical risk factors are urinary tract infection, pneumonia, diabetes and old age. Common organisms are *Escherichia coli*, *Neisseria meningitidis*, *Streptococcus pyogenes*, *Streptococcus pneumoniae* and, in some countries, *Salmonella typhi*. In hospital-acquired infections, the increase in invasive procedures (intravascular lines, prosthetic implants or urinary catheters), immunosuppressive therapy and broad-spectrum antimicrobial drugs has led to an increase in the proportion of Gram-positive isolates, especially coagulase-negative staphylococci, although Gram-negative isolates (*Pseudomonas* spp. and enterobacteria) are also not uncommon. Figure 3.28.1 shows the organisms isolated in a large teaching hospital laboratory.

Clinical features

The clinical features of septicaemia often include:
- fever, rigors
- tachycardia
- hypotension
- confusion or agitation
- evidence of a focus of infection.

In severe cases, the patient may present with circulatory collapse (**shock**) and the temperature may be paradoxically low (**hypothermia**). Acute infections are traditionally associated with Gram-negative bacteria but cannot be distinguished clinically from Gram-positive septicaemia. A careful history and examination may reveal the source of infection and help to predict the likely organism.

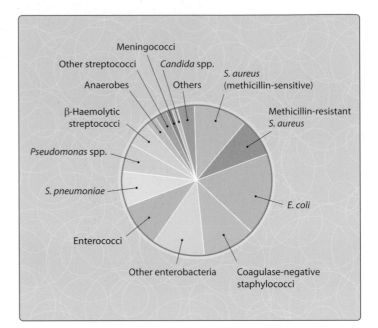

Fig. 3.28.1 Causes of hospital-acquired septicaemia.

Diagnosis

Even in an emergency situation, it is vital to collect at least one set of blood cultures (Fig. 3.28.2) as well as specimens for culture from other sites (e.g. urine, sputum) before antimicrobial treatment is started. Blood cultures are generally incubated for 5–7 days but often become positive within the first 48 h. The first report is the Gram stain of a positive blood culture, which gives some indication of the possible organism (e.g. Gram-negative rods, Gram-positive cocci in chains (staphylococci) or in clusters (streptococci) or even yeasts). This information may indicate the possible source of infection in the absence of clinical signs. For example, isolation of Gram-negative bacteria may suggest a urinary or gastrointestinal source whereas staphylococci may suggest a wound infection, abscess or osteomyelitis (bone infection). The specific identification of the organism (following specific culture and laboratory testing for another 24–48 h) provides further help in achieving a diagnosis: for example *Streptococcus milleri* is associated with abscess formation or infective endocarditis.

Careful interpretation of the *significance* of positive blood cultures is important. Skin organisms such as coagulase-negative staphylococci and diphtheroid bacilli may represent *contamination* following poor blood-taking technique but may be significant in line infections and prosthetic valve endocarditis. Further blood cultures taken from peripheral veins or through intravascular lines, together with a careful review of the clinical findings, may allow a clearer assessment of the significance. Such

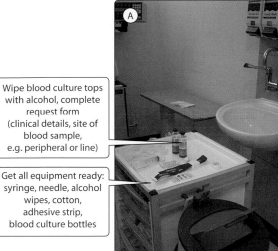

Wipe blood culture tops with alcohol, complete request form (clinical details, site of blood sample, e.g. peripheral or line)

Get all equipment ready: syringe, needle, alcohol wipes, cotton, adhesive strip, blood culture bottles

Explain the procedure to the patient, wash your hands, apply tourniquet, identify vein, wear glove

Disinfect skin site (e.g. 70% alcohol or 2% chlorhexidine alcohol) and allow to dry; draw blood (20 ml adult, 3 ml infants). Inoculate and label blood culture bottles. If other blood tests are required, always inoculate blood culture bottles first to avoid contamination. Place needle safely into a sharps bin

Fig. 3.28.2 Principles of taking a blood culture.

interpretations require close liaison between the microbiologist or infectious disease physician and clinician.

Positive cultures from blood as well as other sites also guide antimicrobial therapy. General suggestions for empiric therapy (agents of choice) are given in Fig. 3.41.1. When **susceptibilities** are available, antimicrobial therapy is always reviewed and modified as required.

Blood cultures may be negative in septicaemic patients because:

- the patient has received antimicrobial therapy
- the bacteraemia is intermittent
- the patient has circulating bacterial toxins rather than viable organisms
- the culture media used are not optimal for fastidious organisms.

Techniques for detecting circulating toxins are not currently available for routine use. Some organisms (e.g. pneumococci and meningococci) may be detected in blood (and other body fluids) by non-cultural techniques such as antigen detection or polymerase chain reaction.

Management

Gram-negative septicaemia is most commonly associated with coliforms (e.g. *E. coli*) but may be caused by meningococci. **Endotoxin** released from Gram-negative bacteria leads to tissue damage mediated by cytokines such as interleukins and tumor necrosis factor. Current research into these mechanisms

may identify agents that could be used to inhibit tissue damage. Toxin-related disease may also occur in Gram-positive septicaemia, particularly with *S. aureus* (e.g. Panton Valentine leukocidin) and β-haemolytic streptococci, especially group A (*S. pyogenes*) infections.

The management of septicaemia requires more than appropriate antimicrobial therapy as well as close monitoring, with particular regard to cardiovascular, respiratory and renal function. Many patients will require fluid replacement, and those with more severe septicaemia may well require supportive management in an intensive care unit.

The typical **complications** of severe septicaemia include:

- acute renal failure
- respiratory failure: acute respiratory distress syndrome (ARDS)
- haematological failure: disseminated intravascular coagulation (DIC).

Prevention of some septicaemia is possible, particularly in the hospital setting. Successful interventions include:

- appropriate use of antimicrobial prophylaxis
- strict attention to aseptic technique and care of indwelling devices
- prompt diagnosis and treatment of infective sources
- vaccination of vulnerable groups (e.g. pneumococcal vaccine for the elderly asplenic patient).

29. Human immunodeficiency viruses and the acquired immunodeficiency syndrome

Questions
- What are the basic features of the HIV virion?
- What are the principles of diagnosis of HIV infection?
- How are HIV infection and AIDS managed?

AIDS is the commonest cause of death in young adults in many parts of the world. The major burden of infection is in Africa, Southeast Asia, India and South America, where heterosexual transmission predominates and the number of cases in men and women are approximately equal. In Europe and North America, homosexual transmission has been responsible for the majority of cases. Apart from transmission by sexual contact, transfer has also occurred by blood and blood products, including injectable drug use, and vertically from mother to child.

The viruses
There are two viruses, HIV-1 and HIV-2, which are accepted causes of AIDS. Structurally, these viruses are identical (Fig. 3.29.1). They are retroviruses, so-called because they encode an enzyme, reverse transcriptase, that makes a DNA copy of genomic RNA when it infects cells; this is 'backwards' (Greek *retro*) to the classic RNA from DNA. The replication cycle of HIV-1 is shown in Fig. 3.29.2. Other retroviruses that are known to infect humans are human T cell lymphotropic viruses (HTLV)

1 and 2, but they are associated with lymphoma and neurological disease not AIDS.

HIV undergoes rapid evolution, with quasispecies being produced as reverse transcriptase makes mistakes in copying the original genome. These are grouped as strains or **clades**, with HIV-1$_B$ being the virus that was first recognized in the USA.

HIV disease and pathogenesis
HIV infects T lymphocytes and macrophages. These cells express CD4 (and other cell surface molecules, such as CCR5), which the virus uses to attach to the cell. Early infection takes place predominantly in the lymph nodes, although CD4-positive cells in tissues such as the brain and gut are also infected. This initial infection elicits a vigorous immune response, which is detectable as anti-HIV antibody after 4–8 weeks. In many cases, this primary illness (or 'seroconversion illness') is manifest as a glandular fever-like illness 2–12 weeks after initial infection. Uncommonly, infection is aborted at this stage, but in the majority there follows a long incubation period with continued viral replication (over 10 billion new viruses per day) accompanied by a large turnover of immune cells. This period lasts months or years, with increasing lymph node activity, which can be eventually detected clinically as a **persistent generalized lymphadenopathy**. As the destruction of immune cells becomes greater than new immune cell production, AIDS develops.

AIDS is symptomatic HIV infection. It is a clinical diagnosis based on the presence of a number of 'AIDS-defining illnesses', usually with detectable anti-HIV antibody. These illnesses are, with few exceptions, 'opportunistic' infections and tumours. There are several international definitions of AIDS, but the most common examples of infections and tumours are:
- infections
  - *Candida* (oral, oesophageal, tracheal, lung)
  - cytomegalovirus
  - *Pneumocystis jerovecii* (was *P. carinii*)
  - atypical mycobacteria
  - persistent gastrointestinal infections (e.g. *Cryptosporidia, Isospora, Encephalitozoon* spp.)
  - *Cryptococcus* (meningitis, pneumonia)
  - herpes simplex virus (disseminated, gastrointestinal, pneumonia)
  - encephalopathy (HIV, *Toxoplasma gondii*)
  - tuberculosis (disseminated)
  - coccidiodomycosis
  - *Salmonella*

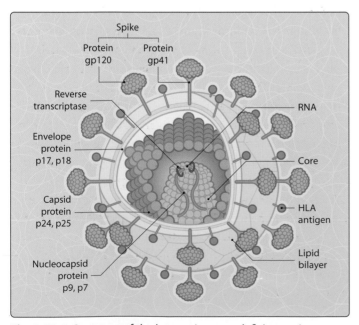

Fig. 3.29.1 Structure of the human immunodeficiency virus.

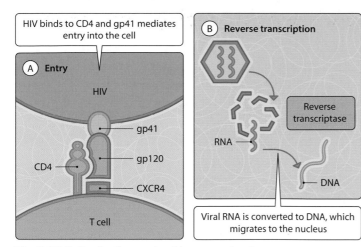
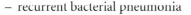

A **Entry**
HIV binds to CD4 and gp41 mediates entry into the cell
HIV
gp41
gp120
CD4
CXCR4
T cell

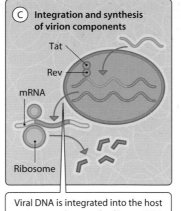

B **Reverse transcription**
Reverse transcriptase
RNA
DNA
Viral RNA is converted to DNA, which migrates to the nucleus

C **Integration and synthesis of virion components**
Tat
Rev
mRNA
Ribosome
Viral DNA is integrated into the host genome and transcribed into mRNA

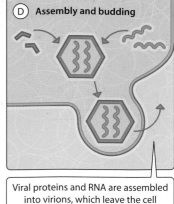

D **Assembly and budding**
Viral proteins and RNA are assembled into virions, which leave the cell by budding

Fig. 3.29.2 Replication cycle of human retroviruses.

 – recurrent bacterial pneumonia
 – severe wasting
■ tumours
 – Kaposi's sarcoma
 – Burkitt's and other lymphomas
 – invasive cervical cancer
 – oral hairy leukoplakia.

Diagnosis

The following laboratory tests are routinely performed for patients at risk of infection: HIV antibody test, CD4 cell count and plasma HIV RNA. HIV antibody testing has been the traditional method for diagnosing infection and remains a useful epidemiological tool. The gold standard for diagnosis is, however, detection of virus by RNA amplifiction, which can also be made quantitative to determine viral load. The CD4 T cell count serves as the major indicator of immunocompetence (classically, reduction to $\leq 200 \times 10^6$ cells/l has been considered the place where HIV infection begins to move into AIDS). Both quantitative RNA amplification methods and CD4 cell counts are used to monitor therapy (see below).

Management

In the early stages, there is treatment of HIV itself, but with the onset of immunosuppression, there is also the management and prophylaxis of opportunistic infections and tumours.

Eradication of HIV infection is not currently possible with available drugs but reduction of viral load leads to improved length and quality of life. Therapeutic management is best with a combination of antiretroviral drugs (Table 3.29.1). Treatment is probably best instituted early in infection when the balance between the host immune system and virus is still in favour of

Table 3.29.1 DRUGS USED FOR HIV

Target	Drug
Binding and fusion (CCR5)	Maraviroc, enfuvirtide
Reverse transcriptase	Zidovudine, lamivudine, didanosine, zalcitabine, stavudine, nevirapine, loviride, delarvidine, abacavir, efavirenz, etravirine
Integrase	Raltegravir
Translation	Antisense RNA
Protease	Nelfinavir, lopinavir, ritonavir, indinavir, saquinavir, tenofovir, tipranavir, darunavir, atazanavir abacavir
Budding	Interferon-alpha

the former. All the currently available drugs have serious side-effects, and treatment needs to be adjusted to minimize these. There is also a continual risk of the development of resistance to a drug, which is minimized by using a cocktail of drugs and emphasizing adherence to the regimen. Postexposure prophylaxis is managed with reverse transcriptase inhibitors.

Viral load (plasma RNA) reduction to below the limits detection of the standard assay (< 50 copies/ml) usually occurs within 16 to 24 weeks of commencing therapy in 70–90% of patients.

Drug therapy is complicated when opportunistic infections arise, as there is a high risk of adverse drug interactions. Management is best undertaken in specialist centres, as this area of antimicrobial drug development is the most active and new drugs are emerging rapidly and being used before licensing.

A vaccine for HIV would be ideal but is beset by the rapid evolution of the virus.

30. Infections of the immunocompromised host

Questions
- What is the infection risk during neutropenia?
- What measures are effective in preventing infection in the immunocompromised patient?

Pathogenesis

The immune system is a complex of innate and adaptive immune mechanisms (Chs 11 and 12). Defects can be primary (congenital, e.g. in complement or the mannose-binding lectin (MBL)), or, more commonly, secondary (acquired) arising from conditions such as HIV/AIDS, chemotherapy, diabetes mellitus and alcoholism. As a result, the patient becomes immunocompromised or immunodeficient and susceptible to certain infections. The type and degree of the defect affects the type and severity of infection (Fig. 3.30.1). Common defects affect the humoral or cellular responses, the complement system and phagocyte function. Complement and specific antibodies are important to opsonize pathogens in order to improve phagocytosis, killing and antigen presentation by cells such as macrophages and neutrophils. The host protein MBL binds directly to carbohydrate surface structures of bacteria, fungi or parasites and initiates complement fixation and subsequent killing by activating serine proteases. T cells are important for the recognition and destruction of virus-infected cells, intracellular pathogens (*Mycobacterium tuberculosis*, *Listeria* sp.) and to activate specific adaptive responses. The immunocompromised host becomes particularly susceptible to pathogens that would not normally cause infections in healthy persons (**opportunistic pathogens**, e.g. *Pneumocystis jirovecii*). Organisms may also disseminate, causing overwhelming infection.

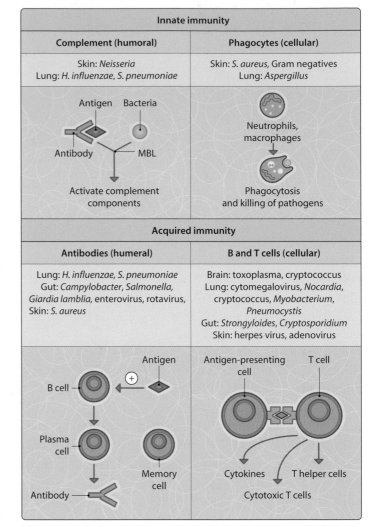

Fig. 3.30.1 Defects in immunity and infection. Mannose-binding lectin (MBL) forms the third complement activation pathway.

Risk groups

Transplant recipients

Patients receiving solid organ transplants are given cytotoxic drugs (glucocorticosteroids, ciclosporin and anti-lymphocyte globulins) to suppress the host's immune response and reduce the chance of rejection. This leads to impaired cell-mediated immunity and increased susceptibility to infections that would normally be controlled. An impaired T cell function encourages reactivation of dormant (latent) viral (e.g. cytomegalovirus, (CMV)), intracellular bacterial (e.g. tuberculosis), fungal (e.g. cryptococcosis) or parasitic (e.g. toxoplasmosis) infections. Patients may present with pneumonitis (CMV, *P. jirovecii*), ulceration in the gut and oesophagus or hepatitis (CMV) or signs of cerebral infections (*Cryptococcus neoformans* or *Toxoplasma gondii*). The patient may also acquire infections through contaminated food (*Listeria monocytogenes*, *Salmonella* spp.) or water (*Legionella pneumophila*, *Cryptosporidia* sp.). The risk increases with the intensity of the immunosuppression and time.

Neutropenic patients

Patients can become neutropenic through diseases causing bone marrow failure (e.g. leukaemia) or secondary to cytotoxic treatment with chemotherapy drugs or radiation (bone marrow transplantation, cancer treatment). Neutophils (polymorph granulocytes) are important in the phagocytosis and killing of many bacterial and fungal pathogens. The risk of infection is greater the lower the neutrophil count ($\leq 2 \times 10^9$ cells/l) and increases over time (Fig. 3.30.2). Patients often do not develop classic signs of focal infection as there are no 'pus' cells to accumulate at the affected site. Fever may be the only sign and should be taken seriously. Common infections are pneumonia, urinary tract infections, oral and perianal infections as well as sepsis. Cytotoxic drugs can cause inflammation/damage to the mucosa (**mucositis**) of the mouth/gut causing leakage of organisms (viridans streptococci, Gram-negative bacteria, yeasts) into the bloodstream, resulting in sepsis. **Gram-negative sepsis** caused by Enterobacteriaceae (e.g. *Escherichia coli*, *Klebsiella* spp.) or *Pseudomonas aeruginosa* are particularly serious and may be life threatening if not treated.

The delivery of chemotherapy drugs often requires intravascular catheters (e.g. Hickman line), which increase the risk of exit site infections and sepsis mainly caused by Gram-positive skin organisms (coagulase-negative staphylococci or *Staphylococcus aureus*) and less frequently yeasts (*Candida* spp.).

If a febrile patient with prolonged neutropenia (>21 days) fails to respond to broad-spectrum antibiotics, an invasive fungal infection has to be considered. Pulmonary invasive **aspergillosis** or **mucormycosis** are life-threatening mould infections that need systemic antifungal treatment.

Splenectomy

Patients may loose their spleen after trauma or elective surgery or be functionally asplenic through an underlying disease (e.g. thalassaemia or Hodgkin's lymphoma). The spleen plays a major part in the immune system as it regulates B and T cell immune surveillance, helps in the production of opsonic antibodies and complement components and removes phagocytosed organisms from the bloodstream. Patients with a dysfunctional spleen are more at risk of infection (e.g. encapsulated *Streptococcus pneumoniae*, *Neisseria meningococcus* and *Haemophilus influenzae*) which can cause sepsis even many years after splenectomy. Patients typically present with fever, seizures and collapse and deteriorate rapidly, leading to death in 50–70%. Malaria and dog bite infections may be more severe. Antibiotic prophylaxis (penicillin), vaccination against the encapsulated bacteria and good patient education are important preventative measures.

Investigations

Accurate clinical diagnosis can be difficult because of unusual clinical presentation and lack of classic signs/symptoms. It is best to culture blood, urine and respiratory samples (bronchoalveolar lavage or induced sputum) for organisms or try to obtain tissue for culture and histology. Laboratory culture results may be difficult to interpret, as the commensal flora, which are usually regarded as contaminants, may be opportunistic pathogens in the immunocompromised host. Repeated growth of *Aspergillus* (a common environmental fungus) from respiratory secretions should be taken seriously and high-resolution computed tomography may be indicated to confirm diagnosis.

Opportunistic pathogens may require specialized diagnostic methods (e.g. immunofluorescence for *P. jirovecii*). For some pathogens, molecular technologies (CMV, *M. tuberculosis*) or serum antigen detection (*Aspergillus*, *Cryptococcus* spp.) have proved useful, whereas measuring antibody responses is unhelpful because of the lack of immune response.

Management

Pre-emptive therapy may be given where the patient is monitored regularly for activity of virus replication (e.g. CMV) prior to symptoms. **Empirical antibiotic treatment** should be given to patients who are febrile and thought to have an infection clinically prior to a laboratory confirmed infection. The antibiotics should be **broad spectrum,** such as pipercillin plus tazobactam and/or gentamicin.

Antibiotic prophylaxis may be given to high-risk patients during severe immunosuppression. Ciprofloxacin is often used during neutropenia to reduce Gram-negative sepsis and co-trimoxazole to reduce the risk of *Pneumocystis* infection.

In highly susceptible bone marrow transplant recipients, exposure to fungal spores may be diminished by providing high-efficiency particulate filtered air (HEPA). Patients should be made aware of the infection risks and how to minimize their exposure to pathogens, for example through food preparation (*Listeria, Salmonella*) and safe water (*Cryptosporidium),* and to obtain medical advice if they are traveling to tropical countries or exposed to infectious agents, for example varicella zoster virus.

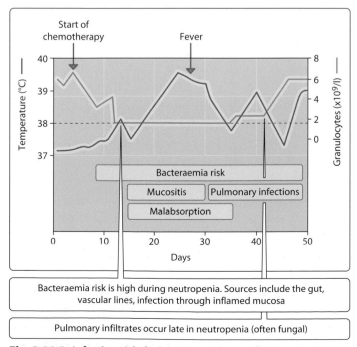

Fig. 3.30.2 Infection risk during chemotherapy-induced neutropenia.

31. Zoonoses

Questions

- What is a zoonosis?
- Which zoonoses are common?
- What are the reservoirs of zoonoses presenting as encephalitis?

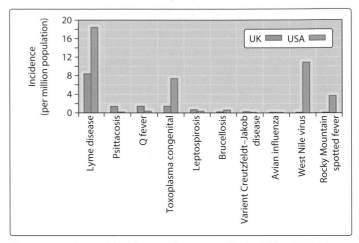

Fig. 3.31.1 Annual incidence of zoonoses in the UK and USA in 2003.

Zoonoses are infections transmitted from animals to humans. They are caused by various bacteria, viruses, fungi, protozoa and helminths. Animals serve as natural reservoirs for the microorganisms and do not usually show signs of disease. Domestic and farm animals are the predominant reservoirs of disease in Europe, and wild animals in the tropics. Many zoonoses are occupational diseases affecting farmers, vets, animal breeders and slaughter house and laboratory workers. When performing investigations, it is important to determine the occupation and hobbies of a patient, as a history of animal contact may indicate a zoonotic infection.

Zoonoses result from:

- direct contact with animals, their excreta and saliva
- indirect contact though food and water contaminated with excreta or saliva (e.g. campylobacter, *Escherichia coli* O157 (Ch. 21)
- arthropod vectors through the bite of an insect, louse or tick.

Impact of zoonoses

In the UK, zoonotic infections are uncommon, and many that were once endemic have declined or been eradicated (e.g. rabies, anthrax and brucellosis) (Fig. 3.31.1). In recent years, many of the newly recognized infectious diseases of humans have been traced to animal reservoirs (e.g. varient Creutzfeldt–Jakob disease, avian influenza, West Nile fever). Factors influencing such events might include microbial changes at the molecular level, such as acquisition of virulence factors, and modification of the immunological status of individuals and populations. Many zoonoses agents such as *Bacillus anthracis*, *Yersinia pestis*, *Coxiella burnetii* and *Franciscella tularensis* have gained new interest because they may be used in bioterrorism.

Zoonoses presenting as fever

Livestock is the reservoir for Q-fever and brucellosis, the latter remaining endemic only in resource-poor countries. **Q-fever** is transmitted by excreta from cattle and sheep and is caused by *C. burnettii*, an intracellular pathogen that induces a chronic inflammation in the liver, spleen, lung and on heart valves. Long courses of doxycycline are required for cure.

Rodents harbour a wide range of pathogenic bacteria: *Y. pestis* is the cause of **plague**, which is still endemic in remote parts of Africa, and **leptospirosis** is transmitted by rat urine contaminating rivers and lakes. Humans acquire leptospirosis by skin contact with contaminated water (e.g. falling from a boat or working in sewage pipes) and develop acute hepatorenal failure.

Birds are the reservoir for avian influenza and for **psittacosis**, which is a pneumonitis caused by *Chlamydophila psittaci*. Bacteria in droppings of infected birds are inhaled.

Cat faeces transmits **toxoplasmosis**. The commonest presentation of toxoplasmosis is lymphadenopathy; however intrauterine infection may cause stillbirth or congenital abnormalities, and infection in the immunocompromised may result in cerebral infection, with characteristic multiple calcified lesions seen on radiography. Serious illness and infections occurring in pregnancy require treatment with drugs such as pyrimethamine, spiramycin and atovaquone, often in combination. **Cat scratch disease** is carried by cat fleas and is caused by *Bartonella henselae*. It manifests as febrile lymphadenopathy, which is self-limiting in the immunocompetent host.

Diagnosis

The diagnosis of Q-fever, psittacosis and leptospirosis is based on serological evidence for specific antibodies. For diagnosis of toxoplasmosis, the dye test which utilizes patient serum to kill viable toxoplasma in vitro is being replaced by specific enzyme-linked immunosorbent assays (ELISA).

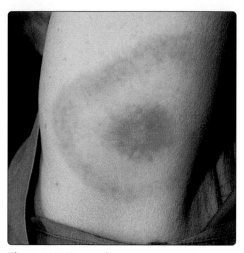

Fig. 3.31.2 Lyme disease presentation as erythema migrans. (With kind permission of the US Centers for Disease Control and Prevention.)

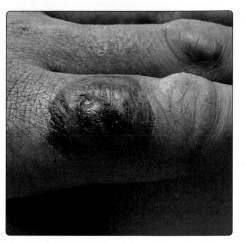

Fig. 3.31.3 Orf lesion. (Reproduced with permission from Spicer WJ 2008 Clinical microbiology and infections diseases, 2nd edn, Churchill Livingstone, Edinburgh)

Zoonosis presenting as skin lesions

Ixodes ticks transmit **Lyme disease** *(Borrelia burgdorferi)* in the UK and in the USA, where they are also implicated in ehrlichiosis *(Anaplasma phagocytophilum)* and babesiosis *(Babesia microti)*. Lyme disease presentations range from erythema migrans (Fig. 3.31.2) to meningitis, cranial nerve palsies and arthritis. If ticks are not removed within 36 h after attachment, a single dose of doxycycline may be given as prophylaxis in endemic areas. Early manifestations of Lyme disease require 2 weeks of doxycycline, amoxicillin or ceftriaxone; late presentation requires 3–4 weeks of antibiotics.

Rickettsial infections have arthropod vectors (ticks, mites and fleas) and cause flu-like illnesses with a petechial rash: typhus, Rocky Mountain spotted fever, Mediterranean spotted fever and rickettsial pox being the best recognized. Serological tests are used to confirm the diagnosis, and treatment is usually with tetracyclines. *Bacillus anthracis* spores are transmitted from cattle by animal hides. **Anthrax** presents as a malignant pustule with generalized sepsis and, if spores are inhaled, as haemorrhagic pneumonia. Ciprofloxacin and, if susceptible, penicillin can be used for therapy. **Animal bites** transmit *Pasteurella multocida* and *Capnocytophaga* spp. in addition to streptococci and anaerobes. Currently co-amoxiclav is the antibiotic of choice. (*Capnocytophaga* spp. are resistant to cephalosporins). Parapoxvirus is transmitted from handling infected sheep (**Orf**) and presents as an ulcerating lesion usually on hands, which is self-limiting (Fig. 3.31.3).

Diagnosis

Lyme disease is diagnosed clinically based on symptoms, physical findings, history and serology. Rickettsial infections are confirmed by serology and *B. anthracis* and *P. multocida* can be easily cultured.

Zoonosis presenting as meningoencephalitis

Rhabdovirus is transmitted by bites from infected dogs, foxes and bats. The infected animal is usually symptomatic. **Rabies** presents characteristically as hydrophobia, which means that the attempt to drink induces a laryngospasm. Vaccination should be offered to travellers who go into rural areas where rabies is endemic. Mosquitoes can transmit **West Nile fever** to humans from birds and **Japanese encephalitis** from pigs. The tsetse fly transmits **African trypanosomiasis** from cattle to humans and ticks transmit **viral encephalitis** in central Europe. For the last, a vaccine is available for ramblers and forest workers in endemic countries.

32. Tropical infections

Questions
- Which infections are common in the returning traveller?
- What are the infectious agents of viral hepatitis?
- Which infectious agents cause dysentery?

Tropical infections are endemic in countries where the climate supports the vector (e.g. mosquitoes for dengue fever) or where sewage is not safely disposed. Clinicians in other countries will encounter these infections in returning travellers or immigrants, who import these infections. Travel clinics have been established to prepare travellers before departure with vaccines (Table 3.32.1) and advice on prevention. Tropical infections may be broadly classified as those causing diarrhoea, fever and skin diseases.

Diarrhoea

Diarrhoea affects more than 30% of travellers during their journey. Diagnosis can be made by culture and stool concentration for parasites. Common causes are enterotoxigenic *Escherichia coli* (ETEC), enteropathogenic *E. coli* (EPEC), *Campylobacter*, *Salmonella* and norovirus, which all induce a self-limiting diarrhoea. Cholera is rare in travellers. The rice-water diarrhoea leads within hours to dehydration and requires intravenous fluid therapy more than antibiotic treatment with doxycycline.

Giardiasis is a water-borne infection as *Giardia lamblia* cysts survive in chlorinated water. Filtration removes the cysts. Stool concentrations are low enough that the parasite may be missed and diagnosis often requires duodenal sampling (e.g. by string capsule test). If untreated, giardiasis can cause a chronic malabsorption syndrome. Treatment options comprise metronidazole, tinidazole, albendazole and nitazoxanide.

Cryptosporidium parvum is a worldwide water-borne infection because its cysts are resistant to chlorination and filtration. Diagnosis can be made by microscopy of modified acid-fast-stained stool smears. Nitazoxanide appears promising for treatment in the first small clinical trials.

Dysentery is a colitis caused by *Entamoeba histolytica* or *Shigella* spp. *E. histolytica* cysts are ingested and release mobile trophozoites, which invade the colonic mucosa. They can transform into cysts, which are excreted with faeces. Diagnosis is made by a fresh stool sample displaying the mobile trophozoites with ingested red blood cells. Entamoeba cysts in stool concentrations need to be differentiated from non-invasive *Entamoeba dispar*. Treatment options comprise metronidazole, tinidazole, chloroquine and nitazoxanide. Except for the last, a treatment course needs to be followed by the luminal amoebicide diloxanide furoate to eradicate the cysts.

Shigella flexneri and *Shigella dysenteriae* cause severe colitis, which in many cases require antibiotic therapy, for example quinolones or azithromycin depending on local resistance. Verotoxin-producing *Escherichia coli* (VTEC) is an invasive *E. coli* causing colitis and is harboured by cattle. Antibiotic treatment is not recommended, because it may induce haemolytic uraemic syndrome.

Table 3.32.1 VACCINATIONS BEFORE TRAVEL TO TROPICAL COUNTRIES FOR ADULTS

Vaccine	Dose	Protected period (years)
Diphtheria, tetanus	Booster	>5
Poliomyelitis	Booster	>5
Hepatitis A	1 dose before departure	10
Hepatitis B	3 doses within 3 weeks before departure	>20
Typhoid fever	3 doses of oral vaccine (Ty21a) over 5 days	1
Yellow fever	1 dose >10 days before departure	10
Rabies (for travellers with wild animal contact)	3 doses within 4 weeks before departure	3
Japanese encephalitis (for rural Asia)	3 doses within 4 weeks before departure	3
Tick-borne encephalitis (for forest trips in northern, central and eastern Europe)	2 doses within 2 weeks before departure	3
Meningococcal meningitis (for Saudi Arabia)	Quadrivalent (ACW135Y) polysaccharide vaccine	3
Cholera	Not recommended by the World Health Organization	

Fever

Malaria is the most common cause in the returning traveller (Fig. 3.32.1). Repeated malaria smears and antigen tests should always be performed.

Among viral infections, **dengue fever** is the most commonly reported one; it is endemic in tropical regions worldwide where the *Aedes* mosquitoes occur. It causes a 'breakbone' fever with a macular rash. Repeated infections can cause a more severe haemorrhagic variant. Diagnosis is by serological test for flaviviruses and treatment is supportive.

Aedes mosquitoes also transmit **yellow fever**, which is rare nowadays since vaccination is obligatory for entry into endemic countries. It causes a severe hepatitis and carries a high mortality. Viral hepatitis caused by hepatitis viruses A, B and E is common in travellers and vaccination for hepatitis viruses A and B is recommended.

Rickettsial infections are transmitted by ticks, fleas and mites and cause fever with a macular rash. Doxycycline is the antibiotic of choice.

Enteric fevers are caused by *Salmonella typhi* and *Salmonella paratyphi* and last for more than 14 days. They carry the risk of intestinal perforation around the infected mesenteric lymph nodes. Rose spots may be seen on the abdomen. Blood cultures can reveal the organism. Treatment with quinolones, ceftriaxone or azithromycin is usually effective but depends on local drug resistance.

Visceral leishmaniasis is transmitted by sandflies or blood transfusions in the Middle East, India and South America. The majority of infections are asymptomatic, but in the immunosuppressed it can lead to swinging fevers and hepatosplenomegaly. A splenic aspirate or bone marrow can be stained for *Leishmania donovani*.

Skin infections

Infected mosquito bites and furuncles are common features in the returning traveller. Itchy eruptions may occur with **larva migrans** (Fig. 3.32.2), which is the hookworm of dogs straying

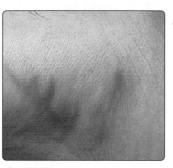

Fig. 3.32.2 Larva migrans (canine hookworm larva creeping in subcutaneous tissues).

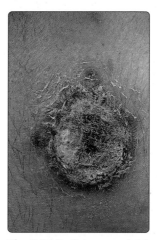

Fig. 3.32.3 Cutaneous leishmaniasis. (Reproduced with permission from Spicer WJ 2008 Clinical microbiology and infections diseases, 2nd edn, Churchill Livingstone, Edinburgh)

in subcutaneous tissues of humans. It is acquired by walking barefoot on dog-fouled soil. **Larva currens** is caused by autoinfection with *Strongyloides stercoralis* (Ch. 34). The eruptions last only for minutes.

Myiasis are subcutaneous maggots of a tropical fly, which deposits its eggs on laundry. The eggs hatch when clothes are worn and the larva invades the skin, where it matures to a maggot within 2 weeks, when it can be manually extracted.

Tungiasis (chiggers) is caused by a tropical flea which invades the foot and encapsulates to produce eggs. It can be extracted with a needle.

Cutaneous leishmaniasis is transmitted by sandflies in the Middle East and in South America (Fig. 3.32.3). *Leishmania tropica* and *Leishmania mexicana* induce a papule, which ulcerates causing a skin lesion for several months or years. A Giemsa stain from the impression smear reveals the amastigotes. Oral azole derivates (fluconazole, itraconazole) can be used for treatment of less-severe forms. **Ulcers** in the tropics can be also caused by *Corynebacterium diphtheriae* (cutaneous diphtheria) and by the acid-fast bacillus *Mycobacterium ulcerans* (Buruli ulcer).

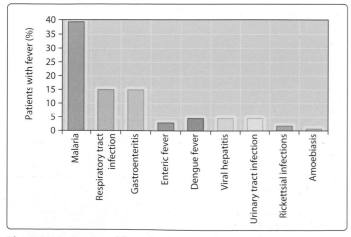

Fig. 3.32.1 Causes of fever in the returning traveller.

33. Malaria

Questions
- What are the different species of malaria?
- In which parts of the world is malaria endemic?
- Which complications are associated with falciparum malaria?

Malaria is an infection of the liver and red blood cells by protozoan parasites of the genus *Plasmodium*. Malaria is one of the most serious health problems facing humanity today, affecting four hundred million people worldwide and causing over 2 million deaths each year. Four species infect humans of which *P. falciparum* is the most common and dangerous.

Life cycle

Malaria is spread by the bite of an infected female *Anopheles* mosquito. Occasional transmissions occur via blood transfusions and intrapartum via the placenta (mainly with *P. vivax*). The parasite has a complex life cycle involving sexual reproduction in the mosquito and asexual reproduction in liver parenchymal cells and erythrocytes (red blood cells) in humans (Fig. 3.33.1). In *P. ovale* and *P. vivax* infection, some sporozoites remain dormant as **hypnozoites** in the parenchymal cells, only starting the process of schizogony months or years later.

Epidemiology

In spite of intensive control measures, malaria remains widely distributed in the tropics and subtropics of Africa, Asia and Latin America (Fig. 3.33.2). *P. falciparum* and *P. vivax* account for 95% of all malaria cases, and 80% of these occur in tropical Africa:

- *P. falciparum*: malignant tertian malaria; the predominant species in the tropics, occurring in sub-Saharan Africa, Middle East, Southeast Asia and South America
- *P. vivax*: benign tertian malaria; common in the tropics, subtropics and some temperate regions, except in West Africa
- *P. ovale*: ovale tertian malaria; common in West Africa
- *P. malariae*: quartan malaria; occurs in the tropics (sub-Saharan Africa, India, Far East).

Clinical features

The repeated rounds of erythrocyte invasion and rupture release toxins that cause bouts of high fever. The periodicity of fever is not sufficiently specific to make an aetiological diagnosis

although the malarias were classically described in terms of the fever cycles. Classic symptoms include:

- cycles of shaking chills followed by fever and profuse sweating
- anaemia and jaundice caused by erythrocyte destruction
- liver and spleen enlargement.

Complications of *P. falciparum* infections comprise cerebral malaria, hypoglycaemia and severe haemolysis. High levels of enlarged parasitized erythrocytes lead to reduced capillary flow in brain and other organs. The resulting acidosis causes confusion, coma, seizures and death. Hypoglycaemia occurs when parasite-induced cytokine release impairs hepatic gluconeogenesis,

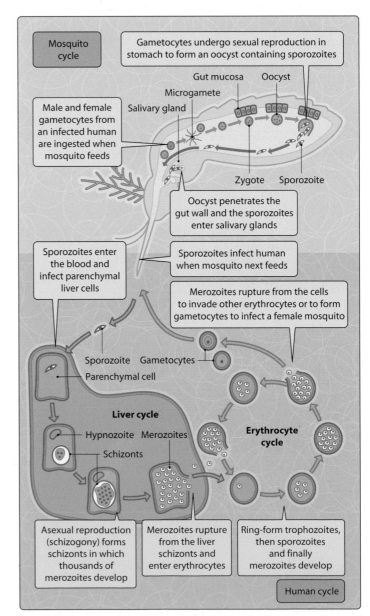

Fig. 3.33.1 Generalized life cycle of *Plasmodium* spp.

which is most pronounced in children, pregnancy and on quinine therapy. Severe cases of haemolysis cause haemoglobinuria ('blackwater fever') and renal failure.

The dormant liver hypnozoites formed in ovale and vivax malaria can result in relapse many years after the initial infection. *P. malariae* can cause the formation of antigen–antibody complexes, which bind to the glomerular basement membrane resulting in nephrotic syndrome.

Diagnosis

Malaria should be suspected in any case of fever associated with travel to endemic areas. Diagnosis is made by clinical history and symptoms and microscopic examination of blood to identify the erythrocytic forms (Fig. 3.33.3). This permits the differentiation of *Plasmodium* species, which is vital in the correct choice of treatment. Dipstick tests have been developed, which detect malarial antigens in blood.

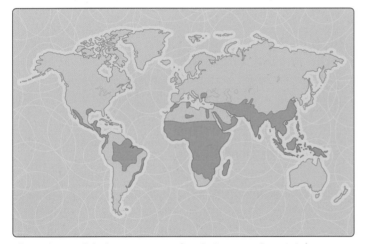

Fig. 3.33.2 Global occurrence of malaria.

Management

Chloroquine remains the drug of choice for non-falciparum malaria. For falciparum malaria, quinine and artemisinin drugs have replaced chloroquine for empirical treatment, because chloroquine resistance has emerged in many parts of the world. Possible regimens include

- *P. falciparum*: quinine or artemisinin followed by doxycycline
- *P. vivax*: choroquine plus primaquine
- *P. ovale*: choroquine plus primaquine
- *P. malariae*: choroquine.

Current advice on area-specific malaria treatment can be found on the websites of the US Centers for Disease Control and Prevention, the UK Health Protection Agency or the World Health Organization. Alternative drugs are mefloquine and the combination of sulfadoxine plus pyrimethamine. However, resistance to these agents is also being reported. Primaquine should be included in regimens for ovale and vivax malaria to destroy the liver hypnozoites.

Prevention

Vaccines are being developed but are not yet available against malaria. Travellers to endemic areas must protect themselves from infection and seek expert advice about antimalarial prophylaxis before embarking. The regimen for drug prophylaxis depends on whether resistance is present in the area and current advice can be found on the websites cited above. Examples include chloroquine ± proguanil, atovaquone plus proguanil, doxycycline and mefloquine. Preventing mosquito bites by covering limbs, using insect repellents and sleeping under mosquito nets is also essential. Stagnant water, the breeding ground of mosquitoes, should also be avoided.

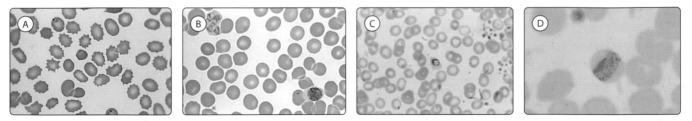

Fig. 3.33.3 Species-specific identification of malaria. A. Malignant tertian malaria caused by *P. falciparum*; trophozoites are small. B. Benign tertian malaria caused by *P. vivax*; trophozoites are large and red blood cells contain Schüffner dots. C. Ovale tertian malaria caused by *P. ovale*; infected red blood cells become irregular and contain James dots. D. Quartan malaria caused by *P. malariae*; some trophozoites form bands in the red blood cells.

34. Parasitic infections

Questions

- Which adult nematodes live in the small bowels of humans?
- Which parasites cause liver pathology?
- By which insect is onchocerciasis transmitted?

The helminths are subdivided into nematodes, cestodes and trematodes.

Soil-transmitted nematodes (roundworms)

The roundworms, apart from *Enterobius vermicularis*, can survive outside of the host and are transmitted by faecally contaminated soil. Their larvae require migration through lungs and tissues before maturing to an adult worm. This migration induces an eosinophilia. Diagnosis is usually made by stool concentration for ova and parasites. For treatment, many options are available (Ch. 44).

Enterobius vermicularis (threadworm, pinworm, oxyuris) lives in the caecum and passes to the anus to lay eggs, which causes anal pruritus. Eggs under fingernails lead to faecal–oral transmission in households. Diagnosis is made by microscopy of tape preparations from the anus.

Ascaris lumbricoides is common in children living in poor hygienic conditions. Ascaris eggs contaminating food are swallowed and liberate larvae in the small bowels, which migrate through the lung to get back through the oesophagus to the bowels, where they remain as adult worms. Heavy infections can cause intestinal obstructions and wandering worms can block the bile duct.

Hookworm (*Ancylostoma duodenale, Necator americanus*) eggs hatch in the soil and the larvae penetrate the skin of the host. After migration through the lungs and oesophagus, the adult worm finds its final destination in the small bowels, where it sucks blood through the mucosa causing anaemia.

Whipworm (*Trichuris trichiuria*) eggs are swallowed with contaminated food and liberate larvae in the caecum, from where they colonize the large bowels to feed on tissue juices. Heavy infestation can lead to dysentery and rectal prolapse.

Toxocara canis **and** *T. cati* are the roundworms of dogs and cats. Children get infected in fouled sandpits in public parks. After swallowing the eggs, the larvae are liberated in the intestines, from where they migrate for 1 or 2 years through organs without final destination in humans. Sometimes larval migration becomes symptomatic as hepatosplenomegaly (visceral larva migrans) or as chorioretinitis or strabism (ocular larva migrans).

Visceral larva migrans can be treated with anthelminthic drugs, whereas ocular larva migrans requires laser photocoagulation.

Strongyloides larva are excreted by faeces and develop adult worms in soil. Their larvae penetrate the skin of the human host in order to migrate via the lung to the bowels. These infective larvae can penetrate the bowel or anal skin and autoinfect the host, causing the characteristic larva currens (Fig. 3.34.1). Immunosuppression can induce a **hyperinfection syndrome**, with peritonitis and Gram-negative sepsis.

Intestinal tapeworms (cestodes)

The most important human tapeworms are *Taenia saginata* (beef tapeworm) and *Taenia solium* (pork tapeworm) (Fig. 3.34.2). Humans acquire tapeworms by eating undercooked meat containing cysticerci (larval cysts in muscle), which gives the meat a 'measly' appearance. The cyst evaginates in the small intestines and attaches to the mucosa, where it forms proglottids and grows to an adult worm of 5–10 m in length. Infection remains asymptomatic until the mobile proglottids are passed in the stool. If humans ingest eggs of *T. solium* with faecally contaminated food, the larva migrates to the muscles or to the brain to encyst, causing muscle calcifications and seizures (**neurocysticercosis**, Fig. 3.34.3).

Parasites in the liver

A **hydatid cyst** develops when herbivores or humans ingest eggs of *Echinococcus* **spp.**, which are small tapeworms of dogs and foxes. The larvae (oncospheres) are released in the small intestines and invade the circulation until they are trapped in capillaries of the liver or lung, where they form a fluid-filled cyst with a brood capsule full of protoscolices (**hydatid sand**). Cysts are asymptomatic for years before they obstruct the biliary tree or get secondarily infected. Under cover of anthelminthic therapy,

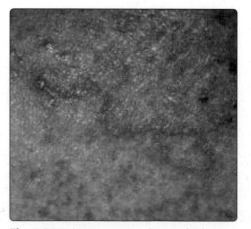

Fig. 3.34.1 Larva currens. *Strongyloides stercoralis* larva in skin; these are visible for minutes.

cysts can be aspirated or surgically removed. If protoscolices are spilled into the peritoneal cavity, they will form daughter cysts.

Schistosomiasis (bilharzia) is caused by *Schistosoma* flukes living in the portal and mesenteric veins. They have a complex life cycle requiring a snail as intermediate host, which produces infective cercariae. Humans get infected when entering snail-infested freshwater lakes in tropical and subtropical climates. The cercariae penetrate the skin and migrate to the portal vein, where they form a pair and move to the mesenteric veins or vesicle–vein complex. They deposit their eggs either in the rectum (*S. mansoni*, *S. japonicum*) or into the bladder (*S. haematobium*), where they induce granulomata. Bladder granulomata cause haematuria, bladder calcifications and ureteral obstructions. Egg deposition into the mesenteric veins causes colitis and portal vein occlusion, with subsequent portal hypertension and ascites. Diagnosis is made by detection of antibodies to schistosomes or of eggs by microscopy of urine or stool concentrations.

Oriental liver flukes have a similar complex life cycle as *Schistosoma* spp but their cercariae invade fish (*Opisthorchis* spp.) or water-grown vegetables (*Fasciola hepatica*). Humans are infected by eating raw fish or water vegetables, and the flukes migrate to the biliary tree, where they cause cholangitis and jaundice.

An **amoebic liver abscess** develops when trophozoites of *Entamoeba histolytica* ascend from the colon to the portal vein and invade liver tissue (Fig. 3.34.4). Patients present with hepatomegaly, hepatic tenderness and a leukocytosis. A 10 day course of metronidazole is usually sufficient to eliminate the abscess.

Filariasis

Onchocerciasis is transmitted by the biting black fly *Simulium*, whose habitat is along fast-flowing rivers in Africa and Central America. The adult filaria lives in subcutaneous nodules and produces microfilariae, which invade all organs including the eye, causing blindness. They cause an itchy papular rash and can be easily detected by microscopy of a skin snip.

Lymphatic filariasis is transmitted by moquitoes in tropical climates of Africa (*Wuchereria bancrofti*) and of Asia (*Brugia* spp.) The adult worm lives in the lymphatics of the groin, causing chronic lymphangitis, which leads to elephantiasis and hydrocele.

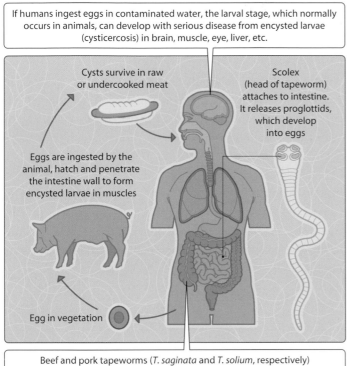

If humans ingest eggs in contaminated water, the larval stage, which normally occurs in animals, can develop with serious disease from encysted larvae (cysticercosis) in brain, muscle, eye, liver, etc.

Cysts survive in raw or undercooked meat

Scolex (head of tapeworm) attaches to intestine. It releases proglottids, which develop into eggs

Eggs are ingested by the animal, hatch and penetrate the intestine wall to form encysted larvae in muscles

Egg in vegetation

Beef and pork tapeworms (*T. saginata* and *T. solium*, respectively) have the human as the definitive host. They cause abdominal symptoms

Fig. 3.34.2 Life cycle of *Taenia* spp. These tapeworms can become several metres long.

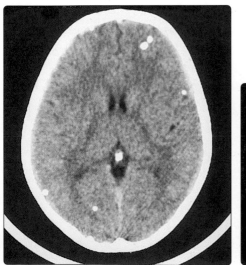

Fig. 3.34.3 Neurocysticercosis. *T. solium* cysticerci in brain as ring-enhancing lesions.

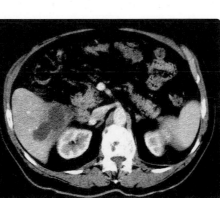

Fig. 3.34.4 Amoebic liver abscess shown by computed tomography.

35. Pyrexia of unknown origin

Questions
- What is meant by fever of unknown origin?
- Which investigations are useful?
- What are common causes?

Definition and clinical presentation

Pyrexia or fever of unknown origin (PUO or FUO) is difficult to investigate because the patients have few signs and symptoms; consequently, the list of differential diagnoses is large and the need for investigation correspondingly greater. Three features define PUO:

- an illness of more than 3 weeks in duration
- a temperature greater than 38.3°C (101°F) on several occasions
- no specific diagnosis after a week of investigations.

There are over 200 reported diverse causes of PUO, which vary slightly according to age. As immunosuppressed patients have a different spectrum of causes than immunocompetent hosts, PUO can be subclassified by type of immunosuppression:

- neutropenic
- nosocomial
- HIV associated.

Investigation is expensive both in time and resources, and it is important to ensure that the patient does indeed have a pyrexia and that it is not a **factitious** fever. Body temperature is normally higher in the evening than the morning, but some healthy individuals have an exaggerated circadian temperature rhythm. Others may invent physical diseases to gain medical attention (Münchausen syndrome), and an unexplained temperature is one means of doing this, either by manipulating the temperature recording device or even injection of contaminated materials.

Investigations

A rational approach should be based on the relative frequency of different causes and their importance to the health of the patient. Every case requires a comprehensive history and *careful* and *repeated* physical examination. History should include a thorough systems review with particular care concerning travel, occupational history and hobbies, pets and animal contact, drug prescriptions and other drug intake, familial diseases, previous illness and alcohol consumption.

A complete examination should include examination of the teeth, ears, fundoscopy and review of the skin in good light for faint rashes. This must be repeated at frequent intervals to spot important developing or fleeting physical signs. Temperature should be recorded methodically, although the great majority of patients never display the characteristic patterns of fever described in the textbooks.

Investigation may include samples sent for laboratory testing; non-invasive tests such as diagnostic radiology and ultrasound and radionuclide scanning; a tuberculin skin test or the more tuberculosis-specific interferon test on patients' monocytes; and invasive testing such as biopsy, endoscopy and surgical exploration. A possible minimum set of investigations is listed in Fig. 3.35.1. Further investigation will depend upon what has already been done, and clues that may be obtained from the history and examination, working through all the possible differential diagnoses.

Possible causes

Some well-recognized causes of PUO are given in Fig. 3.35.2. However, in the majority of cases, the cause is a familiar disease with an unusual presentation, rather than a rare disorder.

Infections.   These are the single most common cause of PUO, particularly in the young. They may be difficult to diagnose for a number of reasons, for example, the patient was taking antibiotics when the sample was taken, the site of infection is hidden or the infectious agent is difficult or impossible to culture in the laboratory.

Tumours.   Neoplasms are an important cause of PUO, particularly in the elderly. Certain tumours seem to cause pyrexia themselves; others may produce it because of necrosis or secondary infection.

Collagen vascular disease. The next largest single cause after infection; there may also be rash, localized limb pain, arthralgia and myalgia.

Undiagnosed.   This category is largely made up of patients who recovered from a benign febrile illness before a specific diagnosis was made.

Common infections presenting as PUO are intra-abdominal abscesses, extrapulmonar tuberculosis and endocarditis. Lymphomas and collagen vascular diseases often pose diagnostic conundrums.

Management

There is no treatment for the clinical presentation of PUO itself; success lies in finding the cause and then managing that condition.

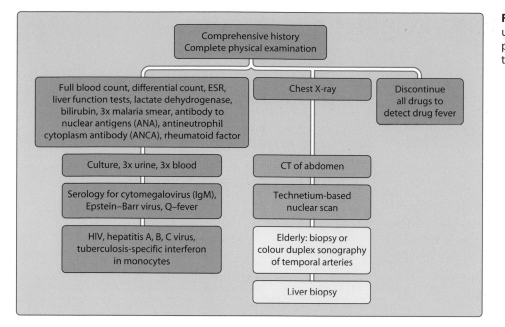

Fig. 3.35.1 Investigations for pyrexia of unknown origin. Red boxes are essential, purple the second set and yellow the third-stage investigations.

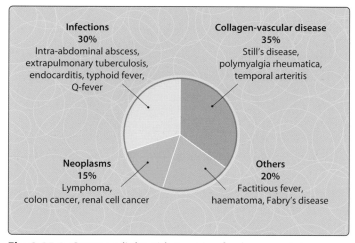

Fig. 3.35.2 Common links with pyrexia of unknown origin.

Fig. 3.35.3 Electron micrograph of a herpes virus.

Febrile lymphadenopathies

The presence of swollen glands with a fever occurs in some zoonoses (Ch 31) and is common in children, where the condition may resolve without the cause being identified.

Infectious mononucleosis is also called glandular fever because of the presence of generalized lymphadenopathy. It is most commonly caused by primary infection with Epstein–Barr virus, a herpesvirus (Fig. 3.35.3). Sore throat, tonsillar enlargement and palatal petechiae also occur with the potential complications of splenomegaly, hepatitis and autoimmune haemolytic anaemia. Large numbers of atypical monocytes in a blood film, the presence of cold agglutinins and a **heterophil antibody** response to horse or sheep erythrocytes, which causes a positive Paul–Bunnell or Monospot test, is also typical. Confirmation of Epstein–Barr virus infection is made by specific serology.

Treatment is supportive. Infections with Epstein–Barr virus may become chronic and it is implicated in Burkitt's lymphoma and post-transplant lymphoproliferative syndromes.

Other common infectious causes of generalized lymphadenopathy are **cytomegalovirus** and *Toxoplasma gondii*. Cytomegalovirus is generally acquired during childhood via saliva, although other body fluids may also contain virus. Infection is more typically silent but, as with other herpesvirus infections, the virus can persist and reactivation occurs. It is a common cause of fever after transplants, and of retinitis and pneumonia in AIDS. *T. gondii* causes a self-limited febrile lymphadenopathy in the immunocompetent host, frequently affecting the neck lymph nodes; in the immunosuppressed, a generalized febrile illness occurs and sometimes cerebral infections.

36. New and re-emerging infectious diseases

Questions
■ What organisms have been recently discovered and what diseases are they associated with?
■ What factors influence the global emergence, re-emergence and spread of infectious diseases?

There has been considerable success in combating infection in the developed world since the middle of the last century, through advances in nutrition and hygiene as well as the development of drugs and vaccines. The worldwide eradication of smallpox was a notable success. However, despite many improvements there are still 15 million (>25%) deaths worldwide attributable to infectious diseases (Fig. 3.36.1). 'New' infections are constantly being described (Appendix, Table A.2), and there is always the problem of established infections becoming resistant to current therapies (Table 3.36.1).

New diseases

Viruses are potentially the most rapidly evolving of all infectious agents and, therefore, the greatest future threat. Bacteria may acquire or generate new virulence genes and become able to cause new infections. Alternatively, the microorganisms may not change but, because of changes in the environment that surrounds us, they may suddenly start to cause human disease:

■ **possible new pathogens**: *Escherichia coli* O157, *Haemophilus influenzae* biogroup aegyptius
■ **changes in the environment**: *Legionella pneumophila*, related to widespread air conditioning; probably bovine

Table 3.36.1 EMERGING PROBLEMS OF DRUG RESISTANCE

Infectious agent	Resistance problem
Herpes simplex virus	Aciclovir
Human immunodeficiency virus	Zidovudine and others
Methicillin-resistant *Staphylococcus aureus* (MRSA)	β-Lactams (and other antibiotics)
Vancomycin-resistant *S. aureus* (VISA or VRSA)	Methicillin; now also resistant to vancomycin
Penicillin-resistant *Streptococcus pneumoniae*	β-Lactams (and other antibiotics)
Neisseria gonorrhoeae	Penicillin, tetracycline, quinolones
Glycopeptide-resistant *Enterococcus* spp. (GRE)	Multiresistance, including to glycopeptides
Multidrug-resistant *Mycobacterium tuberculosis* (MDR-TB)	Isoniazid, pyrazinamide, rifampicin and others
Gram-negative organisms with 'extended spectrum β-lactamases' (ESBL)	β-Lactams (and other antibiotics)
Candida spp.	Fluconazole
Plasmodium spp.	Chloroquine
Scabies	Lindane

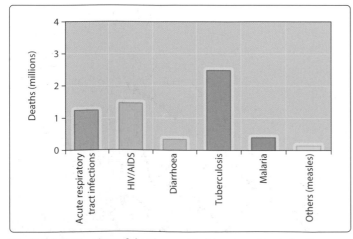

Fig. 3.36.1 Number of deaths worldwide caused by infectious diseases. Source: World Health Organization *World Health Report 2000*.

spongiform encephalopathy (BSE)/variant Creutzfeldt–Jacob disease, related to infected meat
■ **movement of populations**: travellers can take pathogens into areas where there is no natural immunity (e.g. the introduction of measles into aborginal peoples by explorers) or disseminate a pathogen over a wide area (a recently discovered coronavirus causing severe acute respiratory syndrome (SARS) led to outbreaks across the world through intercontinental travel and resulted in a number of deaths).

Established diseases of unknown cause

When the aetiology of a disease is first discovered, there may be a greater appreciation of the significance of the disease, although the disease itself is neither new nor necessarily increasing. There are a number of newly identified pathogens detected:

■ laboratory culture: *Borrelia burgdorferi*, *Campylobacter* spp., *Helicobacter pylori*
■ microscopy: *Cryptosporidium*, *Cyclospora* spp.
■ molecular biology: *Tropheryma whippelii*, *Bartonella henselae*.

There are likely to be many other diseases that have an infectious aetiology that is yet to be identified, possibly even including conditions such as sarcoidosis, multiple sclerosis and bipolar depression. Recent publications have linked an enterovirus with diabetes mellitus.

Re-emerging diseases

The incidence of many infections fluctuates with known periodicity over time, either because of changes in the physical environment, such as the peaks of food-borne illness associated with the warm summer months, or possibly because of changes in the levels of immunity within the population, such as the 9-year cycles of parvovirus infections.

However, for some diseases, these changes may be unpredictable and dramatic. While influenza epidemics occur in October–March in the northern hemisphere and May–September in the southern hemisphere regularly, pandemics, killing millions of people, have occurred in the past and may well do so again. Influenza A virus is labile and minor changes in surface proteins (haemagglutinin and neuraminidase) occur from season to season ('antigenic drift') (Fig. 3.36.2). Major changes (antigenic shift) occur when 'new' haemagglutinins arise, resulting in modified viruses against which the population has little immunity. The possible recombination of human influenza with swine influenza adds to the global threat of emerging infections.

The resurgence in *Mycobacterium tuberculosis* infection worldwide (Fig. 3.36.3), including with resistance to multiple antibiotics, results from the breakdown of public health facilities, from immigration, and also from the emergence of HIV infection, as it has increased the number of susceptible individuals who then form an increased reservoir of infection to be passed on to others.

Old diseases such as anthrax, plague and smallpox have also become a new threat through the increased risk of bioterrorism.

Future challenges, threats and opportunities

As our civilization develops, it is possible to appreciate a number of changes which benefit society but which may also be potential threats to world health from infectious disease, including:

- rapid, intercontinental transport, especially air travel, might allow a problem to be disseminated before it is recognized
- globalization of food supplies: new methods may create new problems, but also, with the increasing industrialization of production, problems with a single producer may affect vast numbers of people
- exploration and use of unknown, potentially threatening, environments such as the rain forest (and, possibly, outer space)
- xenotransplantation and the risk of modifying animal diseases to infect humans
- increasing size and density of urban populations
- increasing migration
- an ever-increasing number of immunosuppressed individuals
- the effects of global warming, natural catastrophes, wars and the breakdown of public health services
- increased risk of bioterrorism.

It is clearly important that there should be sufficient awareness and infection **surveillance** in the population to recognize and to react quickly to any new threat; many countries as well as the World Health Organization have already set up groups specifically for this. There is a constant need to improve diagnostic tools and treatments so that they can be adapted to novel situations quickly and effectively.

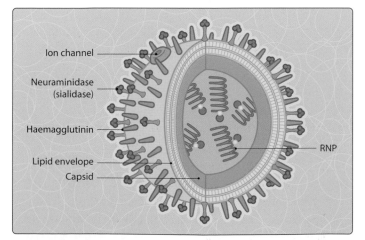

Fig. 3.36.2 Influenza virus basic structure.

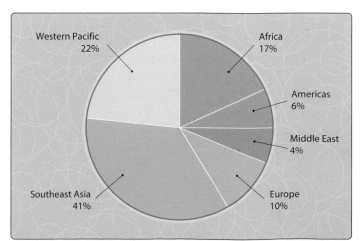

Fig. 3.36.3 Geographical distribution of notified cases of tuberculosis. Source: Global Tuberculosis Control, World Health Organization *World Health Report 2001*.

37. Principles of hospital infection control

Questions
- What are the principles and role of surveillance in infection control?
- Give three different examples of how to control nosocomial infections.

Hospitalized patients are more likely to develop infections as a result of invasive procedures (e.g. surgery), use of medical devices (e.g. intravascular catheters) and impaired host defences through underlying diseases, treatment or extremes of age. A breakdown in infection control practices increases the spread of typical hospital microorganism such as methicillin-resistant *Staphylococcus aureus* (MRSA), *Clostridium difficile* and norovirus.

In England, the prevalence of hospital-acquired infection (HAI; nosocomial) in 2006 was 8.2%. These infections (Fig. 3.37.1) increase patient's morbidity, mortality, length of stay and add to the economic burden. It is estimated that approximately 5000 patients die as a result of HAIs in the UK each year.

Sources of infection

HAIs are infections acquired in hospital that were not incubating or present at admission. **Exogenous infections** are ones where the source of infection is the environment (e.g. via contaminated food, fluids, equipment and air) or through cross-infection from staff, visitors or other patients. **Endogenous infections** are where the pathogens causing infections are acquired from the patient's own microflora (e.g. vascular line sepsis from common skin bacteria). The sources of HAIs and common causative pathogens are shown in Fig. 3.37.2.

The role of the infection control team

In the UK, each hospital has an infection control doctor (usually a consultant microbiologist) and infection control nurses, who constitute the infection control (IC) team. This team produces and implements policies and procedures on infection control and advises on prevention and control of hospital infection. The team monitors HAIs and outbreaks using **surveillance**, which is the systematic collection, analysis, interpretation and feedback of data on specific infections (e.g. surgical wound infection) or alert organisms (e.g. MRSA and *Clostridium difficile*). Regular **audit** of infection control practices against set standards helps to assess compliance with IC procedures/policies and aims to improve quality. The IC team also provides education for healthcare workers on topics such as hand washing and needlestick injuries to increase awareness.

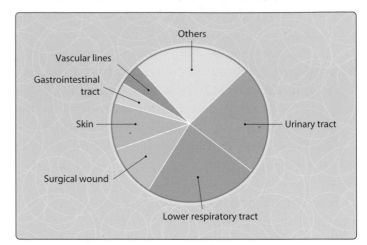

Fig. 3.37.1 Main hospital-acquired infections.

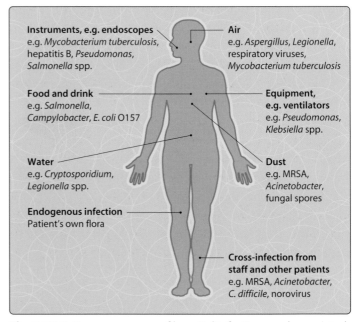

Fig. 3.37.2 Common source of hospital infections and associated pathogens. MRSA, methicillin-resistant *Staphylococcus aureus*.

Control of nosocomial infection

Control is based on three main strategies: minimizing and controlling exposure to microorganisms, preventing transmission and improving patients' resistance to infection.

Minimizing and controlling exposure to microorganisms

Environmental hygiene involves the decontamination (cleaning and disinfections/sterilization) of contaminated equipment (e.g. ventilator tubing) or medical devices (e.g. surgical instruments) or the use of single use (disposable) items (Fig. 3.37.3). Patients need to be provided with food and drinks free from harmful pathogens, clean linen and a clean environment including water and air of appropriate quality. Policies for safe disposal of hospital waste (including sharps) reduce the risk of transmission of blood-borne viruses and other harmful pathogens.

Screening for suspected carriage or infection with certain transmissible pathogens should be carried out for patients (e.g. for tuberculosis, MRSA) and treatment instituted if required. Staff should have health checks (e.g. hepatitis B virus infection) before employment and necessary immunizations. Policies should be in place for reporting potentially infectious conditions (e.g. diarrhoea) or incidences (e.g. needlestick injuries).

Preventing transmission

Blocking routes of transmission may reduce the risk of HAIs. There are three main routes to consider: air-borne (droplets or smaller droplet nuclei), direct contact and faecal–oral.

Fungal spores (*Apergillus*) or skin bacteria (staphylococci and other Gram-positive bacteria) can be carried on dust particles and skin scales. The air-borne route may also spread respiratory viruses and bacteria during coughing or sneezing (e.g. tuberculosis, influenza). Air-borne spread may be controlled by placing the infected patient in source isolation or protecting the vulnerable patient by use of filtered air (e.g. operating theatres or protective isolation). Patients with organisms that pose a risk for others (e.g. MRSA, vancomycin-resistant enterococci (VRE), *C. difficile*) are placed in **source isolation** to minimize spread. If the pathogen is air borne (e.g. tuberculosis), the isolation room should be under **negative pressure**, which directs the airflow into the room to prevent bacteria from escaping. **Protective isolation** is provided for highly susceptible patients (e.g. neutropenic bone marrow transplant recipients). In order to prevent exposure of the patient to bacteria and fungal spores, the room should be under **positive pressure**, directing the airflow out from the room. Staff should wear protective clothing: disposable gloves and aprons (masks if in negative pressure room).

Pathogens can be transmitted by direct contact between the patient and equipment or staff. This route is minimized by **aseptic technique**, taking care when handling dressings, secretions and excretions that may transmit organisms directly by hands or via contaminated equipment (e.g. wash bowls). Any contact with infected or colonized patients (or their immediate environment) may transfer organisms (e.g. MRSA, VRE) via the hands of staff. It is, therefore, very important to apply the appropriate hand hygiene (Table 3.37.1) and technique (Fig. 3.37.4) to minimize transmission of potential pathogens.

Improving patients' resistance to infection

The risk of infection is minimized by good surgical techniques to assure haemostasis, prevention of tissue damage, removal of dead tissue and foreign bodies and avoidance of wound drains. Appropriate insertion and care of invasive devices (e.g. intravascular lines, urinary catheters and endotracheal tubes) are also important. Underlying diseases such as diabetes should be adequately controlled as they are often contributing risk factors.

Antibiotic prophylaxis can help to prevent infections during surgery. Established infection should be treated with an appropriate antibiotic at an optimal dose. Unnecessary use of antibiotics should be avoided as it can promote resistance or other antibiotic-associated diseases such as *C. difficile* colitis. Specific immunization (e.g. pneumococcal vaccination of vulnerable patients) may enhance their own immunity.

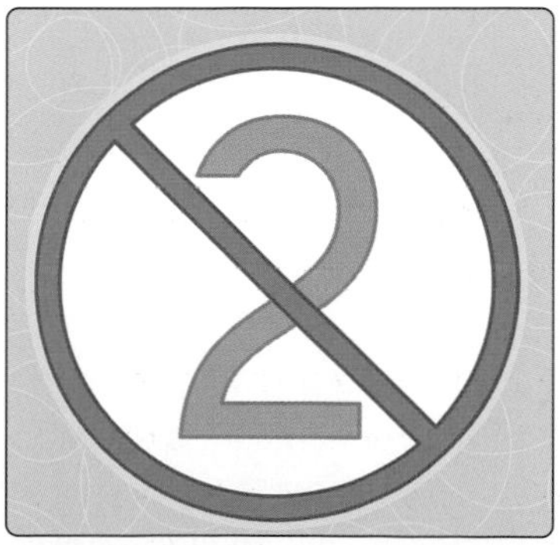

Table 3.37.1 HAND HYGIENE

Technique	When required
Social handwashing Wet hands, wash with soap, rinse and dry thoroughly	Routine duties and before eating Visible contamination with excretions
Hygienic hand disinfection Wash with antiseptic soap or detergent for 10–20 s *or* alcohol handrub (3 ml for 30 s)	Before and after clinical contact with patients
Surgical hand disinfection Wash with antiseptic soap or detergent for 2 min *or* alcohol handrub (two applications of 5 ml, allowing first to dry)	Before surgical procedures

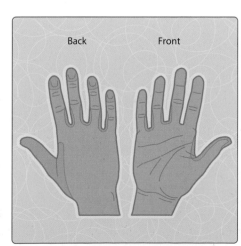

Fig. 3.37.3 Symbol on medical equipment indicating single use only.

Fig. 3.37.4 Hand-washing technique: increase in shading indicates increasing frequency of missing effective cleansing.

38. Sterilization and disinfection

Questions
- Give examples of items used in healthcare facilities that carry a high, intermediate and low risk of infection
- Which decontamination methods should be used at each level of risk and why?
- Name the different methods of sterilization and give examples for their application.

Medical devices such as surgical instruments, endoscopes or other healthcare items (e.g. bedpans, dressings, washbowls, linen) may pose a threat to patients if they are contaminated with potential pathogens, particularly when previously used on infected patients. There are a large number of infectious agents that can be transmitted from contaminated instruments, such as blood-borne viruses (e.g. HIV, heptitis B and C virus) and bacteria (e.g. *Salmonella*, *Mycobacterium tuberculosis*). The decontamination of such items is, therefore, of utmost importance.

Decontamination removes contamination from areas or objects and includes cleaning, disinfection or sterilization.

Cleaning is physical removal of organic matter such as blood, protein, thus physically removing a bulk of microorganisms.

Disinfection removes or kills a large number of vegetative microorganisms, but not spores.

Sterilization removes or destroys all living microorganisms including spores. It leaves medical devices such as surgical instruments free from viable organisms and is recommended for all items that are introduced into sterile body sites or that come into contact with broken skin or mucous membranes. The choice of decontamination method (cleaning, sterilization or disinfection) is dictated by the infection risk and may be defined as high, intermediate or low (Fig. 3.38.1).

Cleaning
Physical cleaning with detergents (**sanitizers**) is appropriate for low-risk items. It is an absolute requirement for items that undergo sterilization or disinfection as organic matter such as blood can protect pathogens from being destroyed.

Sterilization
Sterilization is used when the inactivation of all microorganisms is an absolute requirement. This is achieved by physical, chemical or mechanical means (see the Appendix Table A.5). Dry or moist heat is the most commonly used method in hospitals and laboratories.

Moist heat (steam) sterilization uses lower temperatures than dry heat and can better penetrate porous loads. The most effective and commonly used method is **autoclaving**. Autoclaves are similar to domestic pressure cookers, operating on the principle that water under pressure boils at a higher temperature (e.g. at 15 psi, steam forms at 121°C) that and is sufficient to kill all microorganisms, including spores.

Dry heat (hot air oven) is only suitable for items able to withstand temperatures of at least 160°C and is used to sterilize glassware and metal instruments. Complete combustion in high-temperature incinerators is used for the disposal of human tissues, laboratory cultures and contaminated waste.

Physical, chemical or gas treatment is used for items that would be damaged by heat. Gamma irradiation or ultraviolet light might be used as physical means of sterilization. Sporicidal chemicals, such as peracetic acid, may be used for instruments such as endoscopes. Ethylene oxide gas is a highly efficient method for sterilization but its flammable and explosive nature limits its

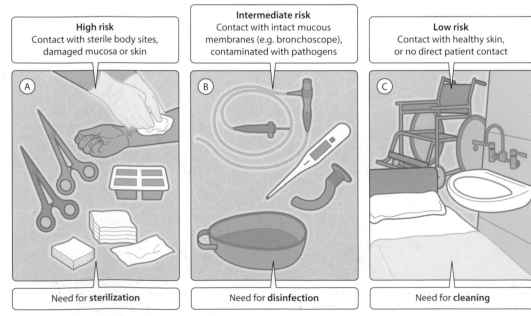

Fig. 3.38.1 Classification of infection risk.

use. Low temperature steam formaldehyde is rarely used because of its carcinogenic nature. Hydrogen peroxide is a safer gas and is a good sterilant because of its highly oxidizing effect. **Gas plasma sterilization**, which utilizes hydrogen peroxide and microwave frequency, produces free radicals and is used for heat-labile items.

Control of sterilization

In dry and moist heat sterilization, it is critical that adequate temperature and exposure times are attained. This will vary with the nature and size of the load:

- thermocouples with chart recorders give a visual record that the correct temperature and holding time were achieved during the sterilization cycle
- Browne's tubes and autoclave tape contain a chemical that changes colour when exposed to various temperatures
- paper strips impregnated with heat-resistant *Bacillus stearothermophilus* spores can be placed inside autoclave loads: spore survival indicating a problem with the autoclave process
- the Bowie Dick test uses a defined wad of paper with a sterilization indicator sheet placed in the middle of the pack to assess steam penetration.

Disinfection

Some medical devices, equipment, healthcare environment (floors, bed rails, wash basin) or hand and body surfaces may need to be disinfected to reduce the risk of infection. Most disinfectants have a limited spectrum of antimicrobial activity, notably the inability to kill bacterial spores. The efficacy of many disinfectants is also limited by their corrosive and potentially toxic nature and rapid inactivation by organic matter.

Disinfectants that can be applied directly to human skin to prevent or possibly treat infections are termed **antiseptics**. Others, termed **biocides**, are used in industrial applications to control microbial fouling and the presence of potentially pathogenic microorganisms such as *Legionella pneumophila* in water-cooling towers.

Chlorine-based disinfectants are commonly used in hospitals and laboratories. Phenol (carbolic acid) has been used frequently in the past but many countries have stopped the use because of the potential health hazard. Hydrogen peroxide vapours have recently been shown to be effective for the decontamination of patient rooms. Figure 3.38.2 lists some common disinfectants and antiseptics, their spectrum of microbial activity and application.

Pasteurization

Pasteurization is mainly used in the food industry. Low heat (63°C for 30 min or 72°C for 20 s) is applied to products to eliminate vegetative pathogenic microorganisms (e.g. *Mycobacteria*, *Salmonella*, *Campylobacter* and *Brucella* spp.) that can be transmitted in milk and other dairy products. It also prolongs the shelf-life of products by removing spoilage organisms, particularly in ultra-heat-treated milk (135–150°C).

Compounds	Bacteria						Properties and use
	Gram negative	Gram positive	Myco-bacteria	Spores	Fungi	Viruses	
Phenolics: Soluble phenolics (Stericol, Izal)							Surface disinfection
Chloroxylenols (Dettol)							Antiseptic
Hexachlorophene (bisphenol: Ster-Zac)							Antiseptic powder or soap
Halogens: Chlorine: sodium hypochloride (Domestos), chlorinated isocyanurates (Presept), chlorine dioxide							Surface, water, equipment disinfectant (corrosive)
Iodine/iodophores: povidone iodine (Betadine)							Antiseptic (skin, hand)
Alcohols: 70% ethanol, isopropanol							Antiseptic (surface and skin)
Aldehydes: Formaldehyde							Fumigation, hazardous
Glutaraldehyde (Cydex, Asep)							Equipment disinfection
Biguanides: chlorhexidine (Hibiscrub)							Antiseptic (wound, hands, skin)
Quaternary ammonium compounds: cetrimide chlorhexidine (Savlon)							Wound disinfectant

Fig. 3.38.2 Antimicrobial activities of common disinfectants and antiseptics. Green, good activity; yellow some activity; red, poor activity.

39. Food, water and public health microbiology

Questions
- How do food products become contaminated with micro-organisms?
- How can contamination be prevented?
- What is the role of public health in the prevention of infection?

Our food, water and air can harbour a number of potential pathogens that cause a range of infections including gastro-enteritis, septicaemia and respiratory infections (Fig. 3.39.1). The advent of penicillin and other antibiotics, or even vaccination, have not been the main factors responsible for reducing the prevalence and incidence of such infections. It is mainly a consequence of the substantial improvement in environmental hygiene.

Food microbiology

Fresh food is easily contaminated by potential pathogens. Vegetables and fruit have soil contamination and even after washing they may harbour microbes if they were washed in faecally contaminated water. Outbreaks of hepatitis A or *Salmonella* spp. have occurred with imported fruit and other food stuff that has been washed in 'river' water or produced with contaminated ingredients. Shellfish pose a particular hazard if grown in sewage-contaminated waters as they filter-feed and concentrate microbes. Some raw meats have been found to contain pathogens such as *Escherichia coli* O157:H7 in burgers or *Salmonella* and *Campylobacter* in poultry, which are often from the animal's gut.

Refrigeration at ≤4°C retards bacterial growth, although those that are 'cold-loving' (**psychrophiles**) such as *Listeria monocytogenes*, *Yersinia enterocolitica* and *Aeromonas hydrophila* can survive and eventually cause infection if consumed. There are a number of other measures utilized to preserve food for longer. Food may be 'cook-chilled' (cooked then rapidly frozen), canned (at temperatures of 115°C for 24–100 min intervals), lyophilized (water removal from food), irradiated (ultraviolet or gamma irradiation), pasteurized (e.g. low heat at 63°C for 30 min), chemically treated (nitrates, organic acids) or preserved by using sugar or salt to decrease water availability.

Although not possible for all foods, the safest approach to preventing food poisoning is adequate cooking, as pathogens do not survive sustained high temperatures. Cooking may be compromised by poor handling so that the food is then recontaminated. Catering services that provide food for patients have to ensure that the food is safe to eat in order to minimize the risk of food-borne infection. Most establishments have a food safety programme based on the **hazard analysis of critical control point** (HACCP), which focuses on areas that are critical to food safety (e.g. temperature control for cooking and refrigeration).

Control of food that is sold is regulated under the Food Safety Act 1990 (and other more specific legislation) in the UK or similar legislation in many other countries.

Water microbiology

Risk to human health from water comes from either potable (drinking) water or recreational waters. Both of these are controlled by legislation in most countries. Drinking water in developed countries is usually treated with chlorine-based compounds so that bacteria do not survive. Surveys have shown that <15% of potable water is used as cold drink; most consumption is with tea and other hot beverages. Illness does, however, occur when there is failure of the treatment process or when local water supplies, such as wells, are used.

Less-stringent standards have to be used for recreational waters including swimming or spar pools and natural bathing waters in coastal resorts. Similarly, most people are not at major risk of illness from recreational water activity unless there has been poor maintenance of pools or water treatment failure. Faecal coliforms are often used as an indicator to measure microbiology water quality (Fig. 3.39.2).

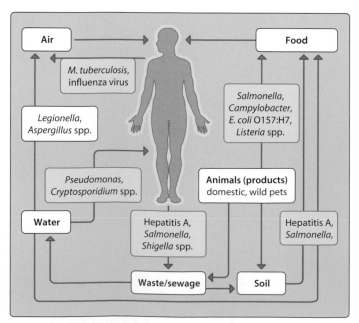

Fig. 3.39.1 Environmental sources of infection.

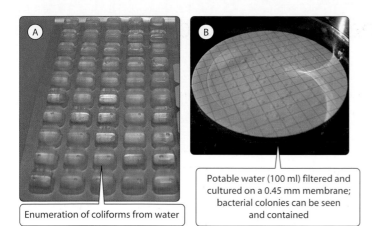

Enumeration of coliforms from water

Potable water (100 ml) filtered and cultured on a 0.45 mm membrane; bacterial colonies can be seen and contained

Fig. 3.39.2 Testing of water for coliform bacteria. A. Enumeration of coliforms from water using special fluorescent media that will indicate coliform growth. B. Potable water (100 ml) is filtered and cultured on a 0.45 mm membrane; bacterial colonies can be seen and counted.

Air microbiology

Respiratory-borne infections are common, and their increased incidence in winter months is thought to be partly attributable to people spending more time together indoors. This source of infection has been enhanced by the use of air conditioning, which allows microorganisms that flourish in the pipework to be spread within buildings. A prime example is *Legionella pneumophila*, which thrives in the warm water of cooling towers and air-conditioning systems, shower heads or spar pools. In hospital theatres, air-borne transmission of microbes is controlled by filtering the entering air. Aerobiological monitoring is undertaken in circumstances of failure.

Public health microbiology

Public health microbiology encompasses air, food, water and waste microbiology. The aims are to prevent and control infectious diseases. Although there are dedicated healthcare professionals, such as consultants in communicable disease control and consultants in public health under the direction of the Director of Public Health (in the UK), many doctors play a role. Prevention consists of several possible components: education, nutrition, hygienic living conditions, good water sanitation, effective waste disposal, immunization and the prompt control of outbreaks of infections.

The effective control of outbreaks of infection is particularly important and implies prompt diagnosis, descriptive epidemiology (including source of infection, route of transmission, and identification of people at risk) and rapid institution of effective measures to abort the outbreak. This should involve an outbreak control committee.

40. Antibacterial therapy: principles

Questions
- How are antibacterial drugs classified?
- What is bacterial resistance?
- How do bacteria become resistant?

Antimicrobial chemotherapy exploits the differences between microorganisms and host cells. Agents that attack targets unique to microorganisms are thus relatively safe to the host—the concept of 'selective toxicity'. Strictly speaking, the term 'antibiotic' refers to naturally occurring products that inhibit or kill microorganisms. It is, however, often used to describe chemically modified or synthetic agents that would be more correctly called antibacterial or antimicrobial agents.

Antibacterial drugs may be classified by their **spectrum** of antibacterial activity (Ch. 41) or their target site of action (Fig. 3.40.1 and Table 3.40.1).

Agents that inhibit bacterial growth are termed **bacteriostatic**, whereas those that kill bacteria are termed **bactericidal**. For many agents, bactericidal activity is species dependent and generally not essential except in some immunosuppressed individuals and in endocarditis. However classification by pharmacodynamic properties, such as concentration- or time-dependent killing, is coming into use for dosage decisions (Ch. 41).

Antimicrobial resistance
A bacterium is considered resistant to a certain agent when bacterial growth cannot be inhibited by achievable serum concentrations of the agent. The **minimal inhibitory concentration** (MIC) is the antibiotic concentration required to suppress visible growth. In diagnostic microbiology laboratories, the disc

Table 3.40.1 CLASSES OF ANTIBACTERIAL DRUG

Target site and class	Examples	Comments/adverse reactions
Cell wall (β-lactams)		
Penicillins (β-lactams)	Benzylpenicillin, ampicillin	Generally safe but allergic reactions
Cephalosporins (β-lactams)	Cephalexin, cefuroxime, ceftazidime	Broad-spectrum: overusage promotes resistance
Carbapenems (β-lactams)	Imipenem, meropenem	Reserved for resistant pathogens
Glycopeptides	Vancomycin, teicoplanin	Vancomycin may be nephro/oto-toxic, assay required
Protein synthesis		
Aminoglycosides	Gentamicin, amikacin	Potential nephro- and oto-toxicity; assay required
Tetracyclines	Tetracycline, doxycycline	Stain teeth and bone
Chloramphenicol	Chloramphenicol	Potential marrow toxicity
Macrolides	Erythromycin	Often used in penicillin-allergic patients
Lincosamides	Clindamycin	Associated with pseudomembranous colitis
Fusidic acid	Fusidic acid	May cause jaundice
Oxazolidinones	Linezolid	May cause myelosuppression
Nucleic acid synthesis		
Sulphonamides	Sulfamethoxazole	Rarely used because of toxic reactions
Trimethoprim	Trimethoprim	Mainly used in treatment of UTI
Quinolones	Nalidixic acid, ciprofloxacin	Early quinolones have limited Gram-positive activity
Rifamycins	Rifampicin	Stains tears/urine, may cause jaundice
Nitroimidazoles	Metronidazole	Antabuse effect with alcohol
Nitrofurans	Nitrofurantoin	Urinary activity only
Cell membrane function		
Polymyxins	Colistin	Used for bowel decontamination or by inhalation
Cyclic lipopeptide	Daptomycin	May cause rhabdomyolysis
	Ethambutol	Visual changes

UTI, urinary tract infection.

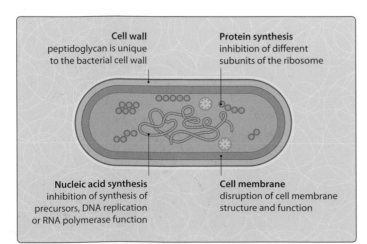

Cell wall
peptidoglycan is unique to the bacterial cell wall

Protein synthesis
inhibition of different subunits of the ribosome

Nucleic acid synthesis
inhibition of synthesis of precursors, DNA replication or RNA polymerase function

Cell membrane
disruption of cell membrane structure and function

Fig. 3.40.1 Sites of action of antibacterial agents.

diffusion method is used to determine resistance, whereby a certain diameter for the inhibition zone corresponds to the MIC (Fig. 3.40.2). Some bacteria show inherent or **innate** resistance to certain antibiotics (e.g. *Pseudomonas aeruginosa* is always resistant to benzylpenicillin). Other bacteria have **acquired** resistance as a result of genetic change. Resistance may result from chromosomal mutation or transformation (Fig. 3.40.3). Spontaneous mutation of the chromosome may change protein synthesis to create bacteria that have a selective advantage and will, therefore, outgrow the susceptible population. Certain species such as *Streptococcus viridans*, *Neisseria* and *Haemophilus* spp. can pick up genes from dead bacteria and transform their corresponding gene with the newly acquired DNA sequence, resulting, for example, in penicillin-resistant pneumococci.

Plasmids are extrachromosomal loops of DNA that replicate independently but can be incorporated back into the chromosome. Those plasmids that code for antimicrobial resistance are called **resistance** (or **R**) **factors**. A single plasmid may confer resistance to many antibacterial agents and can move between species (Fig. 3.40.4). Plasmids are generally spread between Gram-negative bacteria by **conjugation**, where genes pass between bacterial cells joined by sex pili. Such plasmids often confer resistance to many different antimicrobial drugs. Plasmids are usually spread between Gram-positive bacteria by **transduction**, the genetic transfer via viruses that infect bacteria (bacteriophages); here the resulting resistance is generally confined to one or two agents only.

Transposons ('jumping genes') are non-replicating pieces of DNA that can jump between one plasmid and another and between plasmids and the chromosome. They can become immobile (e.g. the β-lactam resistance transposon in methicillin-resistant *Staphylococcu aureus*).

There are three main resistance mechanisms:

- **alteration in the target site** reduces or eliminates the binding of the drug (e.g. erythromycin resistance in staphylococci and streptococci)
- **altered permeability** can reduce transport of the antimicrobial drug into the cell (e.g. in some types of aminoglycoside resistance) or actively pump the drug out of the cell (e.g. tetracycline resistance)
- **inactivating enzymes** may modified or destroy the antimicrobial drug (e.g. β-lactamases, which attack penicillins and cephalosporins).

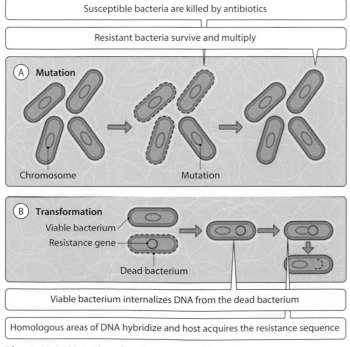

Organisms susceptible to the chemical will not grow, leaving a 'zone of inhibition'

The disc is impregnated with the chemical (e.g. an antibiotic), which diffuses out into the surrounding area

Fig. 3.40.2 Disc diffusion susceptibility testing. A. Organisms susceptible to the chemical will not grow, leaving a 'zone of inhibition'. B. The discs are impregnated with chemicals (e.g. antibiotics), which diffuse out into the surrounding area.

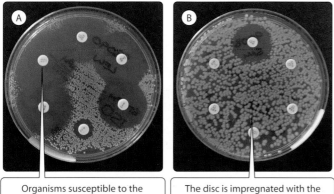

Susceptible bacteria are killed by antibiotics

Resistant bacteria survive and multiply

(A) **Mutation**

Chromosome

Mutation

(B) **Transformation**

Viable bacterium

Resistance gene

Dead bacterium

Viable bacterium internalizes DNA from the dead bacterium

Homologous areas of DNA hybridize and host acquires the resistance sequence

Fig. 3.40.3 Mutational and transmissible resistance.

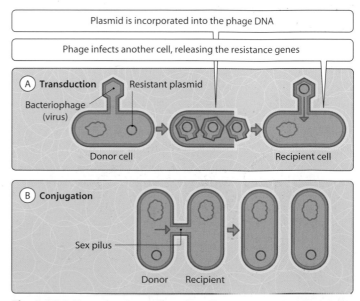

Plasmid is incorporated into the phage DNA

Phage infects another cell, releasing the resistance genes

(A) **Transduction**   Resistant plasmid

Bacteriophage (virus)

Donor cell

Recipient cell

(B) **Conjugation**

Sex pilus

Donor   Recipient

Fig. 3.40.4 Transduction and conjugation.

41. Antibacterial therapy: practice

Questions
- What factors determine antibiotic choice?
- Which is the best dosing regimen?

Some agents are **narrow spectrum** and mainly active against a limited range of bacteria (e.g. penicillin activity against Gram-positive bacteria or gentamicin activity against Gram negative). **Broad-spectrum** agents such as cefuroxime and ciprofloxacin are active against a wide range of bacteria (Fig. 3.41.1). Such agents are clinically useful, but extensive usage is likely to encourage resistance by inducing or selecting resistant strains and allowing gastrointestinal overgrowth with *Clostridium difficile*.

Dosing regimens

Some antibiotics have excellent **absorption** by the oral route (e.g. amoxicillin); others are only partially absorbed (e.g. phenoxymethylpenicillin) and still others are not absorbed at all (e.g. gentamicin). In some cases, non-absorbable agents are used to act against enteric organisms (e.g. vancomycin for *C. difficile*). Metronidazole achieves good serum and tissue levels by the rectal route.

The antibacterial agent must achieve sufficient **distribution** to reach the site of infection. Factors such as lipid solubility, protein binding, intracellular penetration and the ability to cross the blood–brain barrier affect distribution. In order to eradicate bacteria, the antimicrobial serum level must be kept above the bacterial minimum inhibitory concentration (MIC; Fig. 3.41.2). However some antibiotics possess a **postantibiotic effect** (PAE), which delays bacterial regrowth even if the plasma antibiotic concentration falls below the MIC. These antibiotics (e.g. gentamicin) can be dosed once daily and are classified as **concentra-**

tion-dependent killing. In contrast, most β-lactam antibiotics do not exhibit any PAE and have to be given more than twice daily.

Host metabolism and **excretion** may affect the choice of agent especially in patients with impaired renal or hepatic function. Some drugs such as gentamicin and vancomycin have a narrow **therapeutic index**: the margin between therapeutic and potentially toxic concentrations is small. To ensure that safe and effective concentrations are achieved, antibacterial assays are performed. For once-daily high doses of gentamicin (e.g. 5 mg/kg lean body weight), the plasma concentration can be measured 8–14 h after the dose and the Urban–Craig nomogram will then predict when the next dose can be safely given (Fig. 3.41.3).

The recommended **duration** of antibacterial therapy has decreased over recent years. For many acute infections, treatment for 5–7 days is often adequate, and many uncomplicated urinary tract infections will respond to regimens over 3 days. In endocarditis and infections of bone and joints, therapy is continued for several weeks, and successful treatment of tuberculosis requires at least 6 months of combination therapy.

Factors affecting choice of drug

There are now over 90 antibacterial agents available, and making a rational selection requires a logical approach. In practice, many prescriptions are based simply on the suspected site of infection (e.g. respiratory or urinary tract). A more appropriate selection is based on a combination of clinical and laboratory findings, refining the choice by considering specific patient and drug factors, as shown in Fig. 3.41.4. Whenever possible, appropriate specimens should be collected before antibacterial therapy is started.

It is important to minimize unnecessary prescriptions, because all antibacterial usage may be associated with:

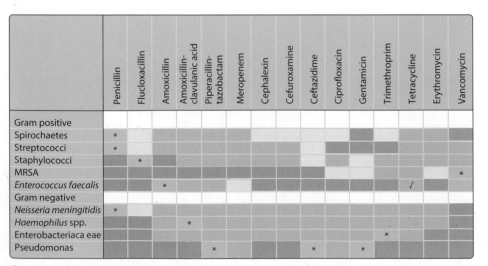

Fig. 3.41.1 Spectrum of activity of antibacterial agents. Green, sensitive (agent of choice); yellow, some activity; red, no activity; MRSA, methicillin-resistant *S. aureus*.

- unwanted effects, e.g. rash, diarrhoea
- increasing costs, antibacterial drugs typically account for around 15% of the drug costs of a teaching hospital
- increasing resistance in both Gram-positive and Gram-negative species.

Antibacterial drugs are unique in that they have an impact on the population as well as the individual patient for whom they were prescribed. Increasing (and frequently unnecessary) use is leading to a corresponding increase in bacterial resistance. Following the significant increase in resistance rates in Gram-negative bacteria, we have now seen a recent increase in multidrug-resistant Gram-positive bacteria, notably methicillin-resistant *Staphylococcus aureus* (MRSA) and vancomycin-resistant enterococci (VRE). This has lead to the fear of a postantibiotic era where many infections may be untreatable.

Rational antibacterial usage can be categorized as:

- initial empirical (best guess or blind) (Fig. 3.41.4A)
- specific or definitive (generally directed by laboratory reports)

- prophylactic (Fig. 3.41.4B).

Most prophylactic use is in surgery with a high infection risk or in implant surgery with severe consequences of infection. There are also a few specific conditions, such as endocarditis prophylaxis, chemoprophylaxis for contacts of those with meningococcal infection or tuberculosis, and after spelencetomy.

In the following situations, it may be appropriate to consider combined therapy:

- for broad-spectrum cover when the pathogen is unknown (e.g. septicaemia) or when multiple pathogens are possible (e.g. perforated large bowel)
- to prevent emergence of resistance, e.g. antituberculous therapy
- to provide enhanced activity, e.g. treatment of infective endocarditis with penicillin and gentamicin.

Such a combination is said to be **synergistic**: the activity is greater than the sum of the individual activities. Significant interference is **antagonistic**.

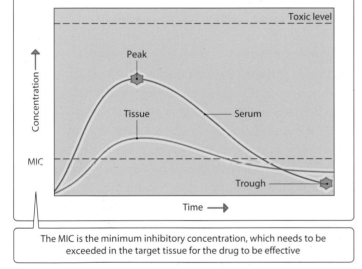

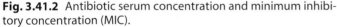

The MIC is the minimum inhibitory concentration, which needs to be exceeded in the target tissue for the drug to be effective

Fig. 3.41.2 Antibiotic serum concentration and minimum inhibitory concentration (MIC).

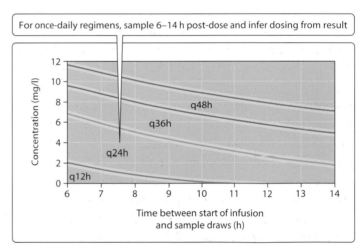

For once-daily regimens, sample 6–14 h post-dose and infer dosing from result

Fig. 3.41.3 Gentamicin monitoring to avoid nephrotoxicity. Nomogram used for monitoring once-daily dosage. The drug-level scale gives the serum concentration.

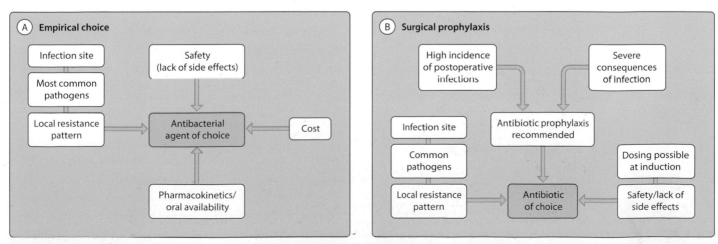

Fig. 3.41.4 Choosing an antibacterial agent. A, Making an empirical choice; B, making a choice for surgical prophylaxis.

42. Antiviral therapy

Questions
- What are the potential targets for antiviral therapy
- What are the available antiviral drugs?

In 1990, there were only five licensed antiviral drugs; in 2009 there were over 40, but mostly for the treatment of HIV and herpesviruses. This is a rapidly growing area but fundamentally the drugs mostly target the replication cycle of viruses.

The replication of viruses depends on utilizing the biochemical machinery of the host cell. Drug selectivity is, therefore, harder to achieve than with antibacterial drugs. There are, however, several aspects of the virus replication cycle that can be targeted (Fig. 3.42.1). Optimal therapy depends on rapid diagnosis, and this is particularly difficult when the virus has a long incubation period or prodrome. Latent viruses also prove relatively resistant to antiviral therapy.

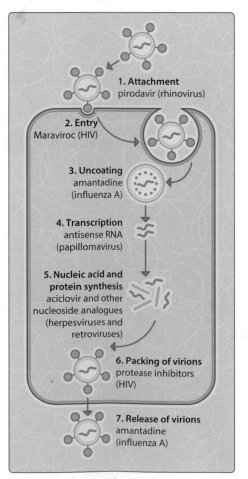

Fig. 3.42.1 Targets for drug therapy in the viral replication cycle.

Treatment of herpesviruses

Aciclovir (acycloguanosine) and its derivatives are the mainstay of treatment of herpes simplex virus infections. Aciclovir is a nucleoside analogue that requires conversion to a triphosphate to be active. The first phosphate group is added by herpesvirus-coded thymidine kinase, which ensures selectivity for virally infected cells. The two further phosphates are added by host cellular kinases to produce an inhibitor of DNA polymerase. The phosphylated drug is also a substrate of the enzyme, being incorporated in place of guanosine triphosphate; however, as it lacks an essential hydroxyl group, it causes termination of elongation of the DNA chain. Two newer derivatives of aciclovir, **penciclovir** and **valaciclovir**, have additional clinical activity against varicella zoster virus. There are a number of agents that are clinically active against cytomegalovirus and useful in patients who are immunocompromised: ganciclovir, valganciclovir, foscarnet, cidofovir and fomivirsen (the last of these is given by intraviteal injection for eye infections).

Treatment of HIV-1

Nucleoside analogues were the first class of drug developed for the treatment of HIV infection and for postexposure prophylaxis. These nucleoside reverse transcriptase inhibitors (NRTIs) act as inhibitors of viral reverse transcriptase. Currently licensed compounds are zidovudine, didanosine, zalcitabine, stavudine, lamivudine, abacavir and emricitabine. Specificity is poor and so all these drugs are toxic: bone marrow suppression, pancreatitis and myositis are not uncommon and may be dose related. Rapid evolution of the virus has also meant that resistance inevitably develops. As resistance to a specific drug is coded by particular genetic mutations, this has been minimized by the use of a combination of nucleoside analogues. Optimal combination therapy also uses other classes of drug that interfere with different parts of the replication cycle.

Nucleotide reverse transcriptase inhibitors (NtRTI) and non-nucleoside reverse transcriptase inhibitors (NNRTIs) have also been developed: the former includes tenofovir disoproxil fumarate, the latter includes nevirapine, delarvidine and efavirenz. They are not without serious side-effects, and resistance also develops to these drugs.

The viral protease inhibitors have been a growing class since the early 1990s and include saquinavir, ritonavir, indinavir, nelfinavir, amprenavir, lopinavir and atazanavir.

There is one licensed drug that targets viral entry, enfuvirtide.

This area of drug development is particularly rapid, and new classes of drug are anticipated.

Treatment and prophylaxis of influenza

Amantadine and **rimantadine** inhibit the uncoating and egress of influenza A. They have no effect against influenza B or C, and their use, particularly in the elderly, is associated with minor neurological side-effects (headache, confusion, etc.). New, less-toxic, drugs (zanamivir and oseltamivir) that inhibit the viral neuraminidase, an enzyme essential for virus entry into a cell, offer therapy with fewer side-effects. There is also the problem of developing resistance with these drugs.

Other antiviral agents

Ribavirin is a nucleoside analogue that has broad-spectrum activity in vitro. Its main use has been for severe infections with respiratory syncytial virus in children, particularly those with congenital cardiopulmonary disorders. It is also useful clinically in patients with severe influenza B and Lassa fever. In combination with pegylated interferon-alpha, it is also the the gold standard treatment for hepatitis C infections. Palivizumab, a monoclonal antibody, is also available for use in severe infections with respiratory syncytial virus.

Interferons are produced naturally in response to viral infection (Fig. 3.42.2). The development of drug forms was hoped to be the 'magic bullet' for viruses. High local doses are, however, difficult to deliver therapeutically, and use is currently limited to the management of chronic hepatitis B and C and papillomavirus infections. Viral eradication does not occur in these conditions, and infection tends to recur when therapy is stopped. Newer 'pegylated' forms of interferon have replaced the standard forms. The use of newer agents, such as famciclovir, adefovir and lamivudine, in the treatment of chronic hepatitis B infection shows promise and may form the basis of better combination therapy of this condition.

Lamivudine and adefovir dipivoxil have also been shown to to be clinically useful for hepatitis B infection. Newer agents such as telbivudine and entecavir also show promise.

Phosphonoformate is an anti-herpes drug that is used as an alternative to aciclovir if resistance to the latter develops, or to ganciclovir in cytomegalovirus treatment. It has an unusual side-effect of causing penile ulcers.

There are a number of pontential drugs, such as pirodavir for rhinovirus and antisense therapy for human papillomavirus infections, that have an effect in vitro but not in vivo. Drug engineering is likely, however, to produce chemical derivatives that enhance clinical activity.

Monitoring antiviral therapy

Antiviral resistance has emerged with the more widespread use of antiviral drugs. Antiviral susceptibility testing methods are now available if clinical resistance occurs, and, in future, antiviral load measurements will be developed. Clinical resistance does not, however, equate with lack of susceptibility of an isolate to the drug in vitro.

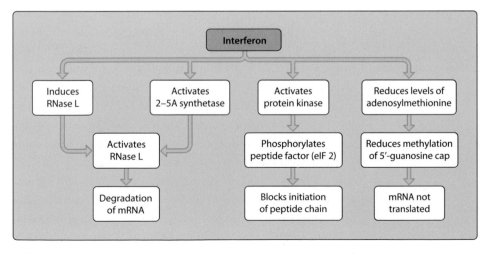

Fig. 3.42.2 Postulated antiretroviral effects of interferons. Double-stranded DNA is also required for these pathways.

43. Antifungal therapy

Questions
- Describe the mechanism of action for three different groups of antifungal agents and give an example for each
- What are the treatment options for invasive aspergillosis?
- What are the treatment options for superficial fungal infections?

There are a number of antifungal agents that can be used topically (e.g. creams) or systemically (e.g. oral, intravenous) depending on the type, site and severity of fungal infection. The choice of antifungal treatment also depends on the antifungal drug sensitivity of the agent (Fig. 3.43.1). Fungal infections (**mycoses**) may be:
- superficial: localized to the epidermis, hair or nails
- subcutaneous: confined to the dermis and subcutaneous tissue
- systemic: deep infections of the internal organs including the bloodstream.

Fungi are eukaryotic organisms and share many common biological and metabolic features with human cells. As a consequence, antifungal agents are potentially toxic to our own cells in their mode of action. This limits the number of compounds available for the treatment of human fungal infections.

As with antibacterial drugs, many antifungal agents are derived from the fermentation products of certain fungi (e.g. *Streptomyces* and *Penicillium*). The principal targets and mode of action of antifungal drugs are through the disruption of the cell membrane or inhibition of cell wall or protein synthesis (Fig. 3.43.2).

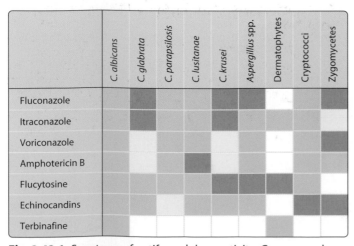

	C. albicans	*C. glabrata*	*C. parapsilosis*	*C. lusitanae*	*C. krusei*	*Aspergillus* spp.	Dermatophytes	Cryptococci	Zygomycetes
Fluconazole									
Itraconazole									
Voriconazole									
Amphotericin B									
Flucytosine									
Echinocandins									
Terbinafine									

Fig. 3.43.1 Spectrum of antifungal drug activity. Green, good activity; yellow, some activity; red, poor activity.

Drug classes
Polyenes
Polyenes are natural compounds binding to sterols (**ergosterol**) in the fungal cell membrane, causing increased permeability, leakage of cellular components and cell death. **Amphotericin B** is the most important member of the polyene group. It is active against a wide range (broad spectrum) of fungi and is commonly used to treat systemic infections such as cryptococcosis, invasive candidiasis, aspergillosis, zygomycoses and deep mycoses caused by dimorphic fungi. However, amphotericin B is potentially toxic and can result in renal failure and allergic reactions. Lipid formulations reduce the renal toxicity but are more costly. Amphotericin B is not orally absorbed but oral formulations can be used for selective decontamination of the gut or for the treatment of oropharyngeal candidiasis. **Nystatin** is also not absorbed orally and because of its toxicity when used intravenously is only used as a topical preparation for ophthalmic, vaginal or oral candidiasis.

Azoles
Azoles are a large group of synthetic compounds that inhibit ergosterol biosynthesis. They are an important class of antifungal agent, being effective in both superficial and systemic fungal infections, while showing reduced toxicity compared with amphotericin B. **Imidazoles** (clotrimazole, econazole, miconazole and others) are used topically for the treatment of superficial fungal infections (e.g. dermatophyte) and vaginal candidiasis. **Ketoconazole** is the only oral agent of this group that may be used for the treatment of systemic or severe mycoses, but it may cause liver toxicity. The **triazoles** (fluconazole, itraconazol, voriconazole and pasaconazole) are effective for the treatment of systemic mycoses. **Fluconazole** is commonly used to treat candidaemia, systemic candidiasis and cryptococcosis but has no activity against *Candidi krusei*, *Aspergillus* spp. or zygomyces. It is water soluble, and drug levels are high in the urine and cerebrospinal fluid. **Itraconazole** is a lipophilic (fat-soluble) agent used for the treatment of superficial, subcutaneous and systemic infections, including aspergillosis. Newer azole classes with a broader spectrum of activity have recently come on the market: **Voriconazole** is being used to treat invasive aspergillosis (including brain infections), fusariosis and fluconazole-resistant *Candida* infections but is not active against zygomyces; the activity of **posaconazole** is similar to voriconazole but it has additional activity against zygomyces species.

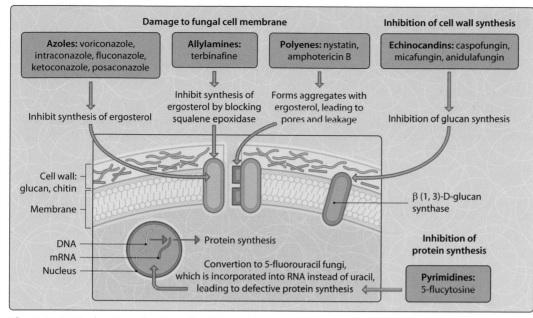

Fig. 3.43.2 Mechanism of action of antifungal drugs.

Echinocandins

The echinocandins (caspofungin, micafungin, anidulafungin) belong to a novel class of antifungal agents with a unique mode of action. These semisynthetic compounds weaken the fungal cell wall by inhibiting glucan synthase, thus interfering with glucan production. The drugs are well tolerated and used for the treatment of serious invasive candidiasis (including infections caused by azole-resistant strains) and aspergillosis. The compounds also show some activity against *Pneumocystis jirovecii* and may be a future alternative to the established treatment with co-trimoxazole or pentamidine. Echinocandins are not effective against cryptococci or moulds such as zygomyces. The poor penetration into the brain may limit its use for CNS infections.

Pyrimidines

Pyrimidines include the synthetic analogue **flucytosine (5-fluorocytosine)**, which is converted to 5-fluorouracil within the fungus and becomes incorporated into RNA, thus causing abnormalities in protein synthesis. Although rarely used these days because of its myelosuppressive toxicity, it may be combined with amphotericin B or fluconazole for the treatment of cryptococcosis and invasive candidiasis (e.g. endocarditis, peritonitis, pancrcatitis, meningitis).

Benzofurans

The benzofurans act principally through the inhibition of cellular microtubule formation, thus preventing mitosis (cell division). **Griseofulvin** concentrates in the stratum corneum of the skin after oral administration and hence treats dermatophyte infections of the skin but also the hair and nail.

Allyamines

Allyamines are synthetic agents that act on fungal ergosterol synthesis. **Terbinafine** can be administered orally or topically to treat dermatophyte skin infections and superficial candidiasis. The drug accumulates in keratin even after the treatment is discontinued, which makes it a useful treatment for persistent (refractory) toenail infections.

Ointments and tinctures for superficial fungal infections

Amorolfine nail lacquer might be used for mild fungal nail infections or as cream for skin infections. Benzoic acid-containing ointments (Whitfield's ointment) can be used for 'ringworm' (tinea) infections of the skin. Athlete's foot is commonly treated with formulations containing undecenoic acid or tolnaftate.

44. Antiprotozoal and anthelminthic therapy

Questions
- Why is the choice of antiparasitic drugs limited?
- Which is the drug of choice for *Echinococcus* cysts?
- Which antiparasitic drug has activity against *Cryptosporidium parvum?*

Recent years have seen many advances in parasitology, particularly antimalarial agents. However, the treatment of many infections remains unsatisfactory. Effective therapeutic agents are limited and of disappointing activity for several reasons:
- similarities between parasite and humans cells can result in drug side-effects
- drugs may not be active against all biological forms of an organism (cyst and eggs are particularly resistant)
- parasites may be in sites that are harder for drugs to access
- drug resistance has limited the effectiveness of many agents, particularly in malaria.

Antimalarial agents
The choice of the correct agent to treat malaria is essential and is based on clinical history, symptoms and examination of blood films (see Ch. 33).

Quinine, a quinolinemethanol of the bark of the chinchoa tree, is active against the erythrocytic stages of *Plasmdium falciparum*, but not its gametocytes. It causes cinchoism (tinnitus, nausea and headaches), hypoglycaemia and sometimes arrhythmias. It has become the first-line treatment for falciparum malaria, because resistance is very rare.

Artemisins are extracts of the qinghaosu plant and are available as intravenous artesunate, intramuscular artemether and as an oral combination with lumefantrin. It is active against all stages of all plasmodial species and reduces parasite counts rapidly. It is used for patients with falciparum malaria in whom quinine is contraindicated.

Chloroquine, a 4-aminoquinoline, is active against trophozoites and gametocytes of all plasmodial species, but not against schizonts and hypnozoites. Resistance has developed in many holoendemic countries. It has also activity against *Entamoeba histolytica*.

Mefloquine, a 4-quinolinemethanol, is active against the erythrocytic stages of all plasmodial species. It has also antibacterial and antifungal activity. Chloroquine-resistant strains remain sensitive, whereas there is cross-resistance with quinine. Psychotropic side-effects are reported in 1:1500 treatments. It is used for malaria prophylaxis and also for cutaneous leishmaniasis.

Primaquine, an 8-aminoquinolone, is active against the hepatic stages of *P. vivax* and *P. ovale* and against gametocytes. It induces haemolysis in those with glucose-6-phosphate dehydrogenase deficiency. It is used in combination with chloroquine for non-falciparum malaria.

Atovaquone, a hydroxynaphthoquinone, is active against all stages of *P. falciparum*, *Toxoplasma gondii*, *Babesia* sp. and *Pneumocystis jirovecii*. It is used as third-line treatment for *P. jirovecii* pneumonia (was known as *P. carinii* and hence the pneumonia is referred to as PCP) and in combination with proguanil for malaria prophylaxis.

Agents against intestinal protozoa
Metronidazole is one of the nitroimidazole antibiotics active only against anaerobic organisms. It is highly effective in the treatment of amoebiasis with *E. histolytica*, trichomoniasis and giardiasis. Metronidazole is less effective against the cyst form of *E. histolytica*, and alternative agents such as **diloxanide furoate** are used to treat asymptomatic cyst excretors. It is also used to treat anaerobic bacterial infections. Inside the organism it is reduced to the active form, producing DNA damage. The related compound **tinidazole** is more effective against these protozoa.

Nitazoxanide, a nitroheterocycle with a salicylic ring, is an oral broad-spectrum antiprotozoal agent with additional activities against intestinal helminths and anaerobic bacteria. Its structure suggests that it may interfere with the host cell signaling pathway, impeding parasitic intracellular replication. It is one of the few drugs with activity against *Cryptosporidium parvum* and microsporidiasis.

Agents against trypanosomal infections
Melarsoprol is a trivalent arsenical active against African trypanosomiasis ('sleeping sickness'). It is thought to inhibit parasite pyruvate kinase and possibly other enzymes involved in glycolysis. Melarsoprol crosses the blood–brain barrier and is, therefore, effective in late-stage disease when the trypanosomes have infected the CNS. As it can cause a reactive arsenic encephalopathy, the less toxic **eflornithine** is preferred for *Trypanosoma brucei gambiense* CNS infections.

Pentamidine is a diamidine compound used in the early stages of African trypanosomiasis, some forms of leishmaniasis and PCP. It is thought to act by interacting with parasite DNA (particularly kinetoplast DNA of *Trypanosoma* and *Leishmania* spp.), preventing cell division.

Nifurtimox is a nitrofuran active against American trypanosomiasis (Chagas' disease) in the acute phase of infection. It acts by forming toxic oxygen radicals within the parasite. As it is neurotoxic, the nitroimidazole derivative **benznidazole** is used as an alternative treatment.

Agents against leishmaniasis

Pentavalent antimony compounds (**stibogluconate** and **meglumine antimonate**) are used to treat leishmaniasis. However, sensitivity varies among species and geographic location. Their mode of action is uncertain but they are thought to affect parasite metabolism.

Amphotericin B is an antifungal agent active against *Leishmania* sp. and is used as an alternative to the antimonial compounds in the treatment of leishmaniasis. It is thought to alter parasite surface membrane permeability, causing leakage of intracellular components.

Anthelminthic agents

Figure 3.44.1 shows the agents available for the various helminth infections.

Intestinal nematodes

Mebendazole is a synthetic benzimidazole that is poorly absorbed and, therefore, is active against intestinal nematodes: hookworms, ascariasis, enterobiasis and trichiuriasis. It acts by selectively binding to helminthic tubulin, preventing microtubule assembly. This results in parasite immobilization and death.

Tissue nematodes

Ivermectin has replaced **diethylcarbamazine** in the treatment of the microfilariae because of reduced toxicity. It is a macrolytic lactone that blocks the parasite neurotransmitter gamma-aminobutyric acid, preventing nerve signalling and resulting in paralysis. The introduction of ivermectin has been a major advance in the treatment of onchocerciasis. It has also been shown to have good activity against nematodes and is increasingly being used in the treatment of strongyloidiasis and scabies.

Albendazole is currently the only benzimidazole carbamate that is well absorbed and achieves therapeutic tissue levels. It is used to treat tissue stages of helminths such as larva migrans, strongyloidiasis, echinococci and microfilariae.

Tapeworms

Praziquantel is an isoquinoline derivative active against trematodes (flukes) and cestodes (tapeworms). It causes increased cell permeability to calcium ions, resulting in contraction and paralysis. In schistosomiasis, the trematodes are then swept to the liver where they are attacked by phagocytes. With cestodes, the tapeworm detaches from the gut wall and is expelled with the faeces.

Niclosamide is also used in the treatment of adult tapeworms, although praziquantel is preferred as it is active against both larvae and adults of *Taenia solium* (pork tapeworm) and may prevent cysticercosis autoinfection.

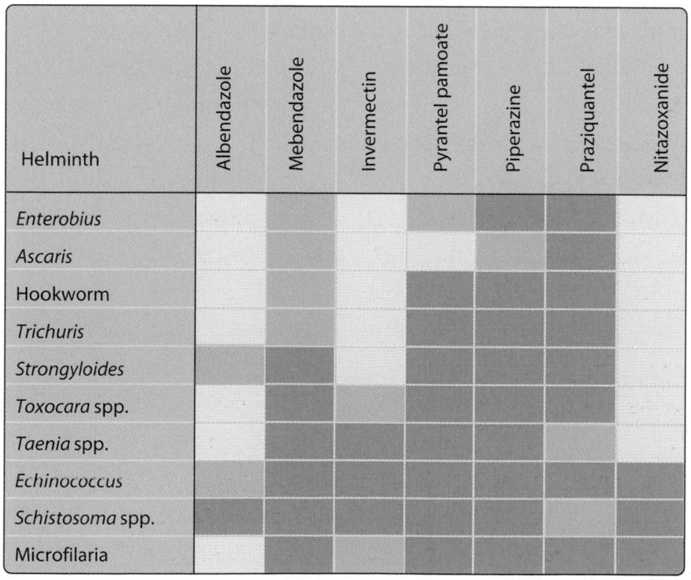

Helminth	Albendazole	Mebendazole	Invermectin	Pyrantel pamoate	Piperazine	Praziquantel	Nitazoxanide
Enterobius							
Ascaris							
Hookworm							
Trichuris							
Strongyloides							
Toxocara spp.							
Taenia spp.							
Echinococcus							
Schistosoma spp.							
Microfilaria							

Fig. 3.44.1 Antiparasitic drugs active against helminths. Green, agents of choice; yellow, some activity's red, no activity.

45. Immunization

Questions
- What is the difference between passive and active immunization?
- Why do infants respond poorly to polysaccharide vaccines?

When Edward Jenner demonstrated, in 1796, that inoculation with material from cowpox-infected tissue could protect against subsequent exposure to smallpox, the science of immunization was born; preparations that induce immunity are now commonly known as **vaccines**, derived from the name of the cowpox agent (the **vaccinia** virus). Vaccines are important against diseases that may have serious consequences and where treatments are less than optimal, particularly when infection is common. The decline in cases of whooping cough coincided with the introduction of the pertussis vaccine in the 1950s, but notifications rose again when fears over safety of the vaccine led to decreased uptake in the 1970s.

Adaptive immunity may be produced by two methods: passive and active immunization.

Passive immunization. Immunity is produced by giving preparations of specific antibody collected from individuals convalescing from infection or after immunization (hyperimmune immunoglobulin), or human normal immunoglobulin from pooled blood donor plasma if the infectious agent is prevalent. Passive immunization may be given as postexposure prophylaxis against tetanus, hepatitis B, diphtheria, rabies and chickenpox.

Active immunization. The administration of vaccines will induce a response from the host's own immune system. It is the most powerful method, effective against a wide range of pathogens (Table 3.45.1; see also Appendix Table A.5)

and is used routinely in many parts of the world including the UK.

Vaccine design

Historically, vaccines have been produced by inactivating the infectious agent or else attenuating it by multiple passages through a non-human host. Some work through a T helper type 2 response to stimulate the production of antibody, for example against the pathogen's adhesins or toxin-binding regions; even the low levels of antibody found years later are sufficient either to abort the infection or prevent severe disease. In this context, it may be particularly important to induce mucosal antibody. Vaccines that increase cell-mediated immunity promote a T helper type 1 response, producing memory T cells that will respond more rapidly and effectively on subsequent exposure to the pathogen.

Many vaccines such as the conventional **pneumococcal vaccine** are based on carbohydrate antigens that stimulate B cells without the help of antigen-presenting cells or T cells. This is a problem for children under the age of 2 years as they have immature B cell immunity, resulting in a poor response to carbohydrate antigens. Newer vaccines conjugate the polysaccharide antigens with a protein such as tetanus in order to get a sustained T cell-dependent response (e.g. conjugated pneumococcal vaccine).

Vaccines often require oily adjuvants that non-specifically boost the immune response at the injection site. However, now that more is understood about the way that vaccines work, those currently under development will be engineered using molecular biological techniques so that they direct the immune response in the manner appropriate to each agent; they should be more immunogenic, have fewer side-effects and be less likely to revert

Table 3.45.1 UK VACCINE SCHEDULE FOR CHILDREN

Vaccine	Age given						
	2 months	3 months	4 months	12 months	13 months	3–5 years	13–18 years
DTP	+	+	+			+	TP+
IPV	+	+	+			+	+
Hib	+	+	+	+			
PCV	+		+		+		
MenC		+	+	+			
MMR					+	+	
HPV							+

DTP, diphtheria, tetanus and pertussis; TP, tetanus and pertussis only; IPV, inactivated polio vaccine; Hib, Haemophilus influenzae; PCV, pneumococcal conjugate; MenC, meningitis C; MMR, measles mumps and rubella; HPV, human papillomavirus.

to the harmful wild type than traditional vaccines. Simple DNA vaccines are effective because the host cell takes up free DNA, expresses it and so induces an immune response against the foreign protein(s).

Problems with vaccines

The **adverse effects** that might be expected after immunization depend on which vaccine was given, but local pain and inflammation, headache, malaise and temperature (even febrile convulsions) are reasonably common. Serious problems, such as encephalopathy, are extremely rare and certainly less than the morbidity or mortality that might be expected from natural infection. Contrary to popular belief, there are few contraindications to vaccination: it is not recommended for those with a significant acute infection or with hypersensitivity to the same vaccine previously; *some* live vaccines are contraindicated in the immunocompromised; almost all are contraindicated in pregnancy. Very rarely, a vaccine such as oral polio will revert back towards the wild virus and may cause disease in susceptible contacts.

While the goal of immunization is the protection of the vaccinated, it also has implications for the whole population (Fig. 3.45.1). If immunization produces high levels of **herd immunity**, infection cannot spread, and a small number of susceptible individuals will be safe; if herd immunity is maintained by global immunization together with case isolation, a solely human virulent pathogen may be eradicated, as happened with smallpox. As the number of vaccine failures or refusers slowly builds up, a critical point is reached when infection can again spread widely. However, many susceptible individuals will now be relatively old and, therefore, the frequency of severe complications is much increased compared with the pattern of disease prior to the introduction of vaccination.

The quality control of vaccine production must be flawless; if a pathogen is incompletely inactivated or a vaccine becomes contaminated, the consequences may be disastrous.

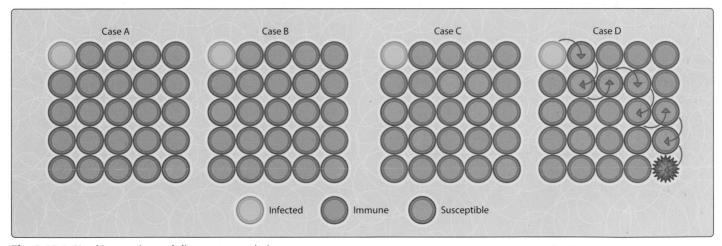

Fig. 3.45.1 Herd immunity and disease transmission.

46. Oral microbiology

Questions
- Give two clinical examples of systemic infections caused by oral bacteria
- What is the pathogenesis of dental decay?

Oral microbiology has been placed at the end of Section 3 as it encompasses many of the areas discussed above.

The oral cavity harbors a number of microorganisms, which form the normal human oral microflora (e.g. viridans streptococci, anaerobic bacteria such as *Fusobaterium* spp, coagulase-negative staphylococci, *Moraxella*, *Neisseria*, *Candida* spp., herpesviruses). Most of the time bacteria, fungi and viruses live in a fine balance together without causing disease. Some people are **asymptomatic carriers** of potential pathogens such as *Staphylococcus aureus* or *Streptococcus pneumoniae* without causing harm. Oral disease can occur if the microbial flora or the host defences change. This may be as a result of hormonal changes, poor dental hygiene, immunosupression (e.g. HIV), stress or use of broad-spectrum antibiotics. There are also a number of systemic infectious diseases that manifest in the oral cavity (Table 3.46.1).

Dental plaques and caries
Teeth have a hard protective layer of enamel. Food can collect in pits and cervices of the teeth, encouraging bacterial colonization and growth, which initiates the development of dental plaque. Within the plaque, bacteria form primitive communication systems (**biofilms**) where they are protected from the host response and the effect of antimicrobial agents (e.g. antibiotics, disinfectants) (Fig. 3.46.1).

Pathogenesis
The bacterial group *Streptococcus mutans* plays a major part in the pathogenesis of dental decay (Fig. 3.46.2). *S. mutans* colonizes the human mouth from the age of 6 months. The bacteria produce enzymes (glycosyl transferase) that promote further attachment of bacteria and food stuff (via sticky dextran) to the tooth surface in dental plaques as well as causing local demineralization (dissolution of enamel) by lowering the pH. This leads to dental caries (Fig. 3.46.3). Complications such as pain and dental abscesses can occur.

Prevention
Saliva has some properties that counteract dental decay. The presence of active antimicrobial agents (e.g. lysozyme, lactoferrin,

Table 3.46.1 SYSTEMIC INFECTIOUS DISEASE WITH ORAL MANIFESTATION

Infection	Oral manifestation
Scarlet fever (*Streptococcus pyrogenes*)	'Strawberry tongue' (white tongue with red papillae)
Syphilis (*Treponema pallidum*)	
Primary infection	Painless, small nodules and ulcers
Secondary infection	Shallow, 'snail-track' ulcers
Tertiary infection	'Gumma', painless, punched out ulcers
Congenital	Hutchinson's teeth (peg shaped teeth, notch in upper incisors)
Valley fever (fungal, *Coccidioides immitis*)	Oral ulcers
Hand, food and mouth disease (coxsackie virus)	Pharyngeal ulcers
Chicken pox (varicella zoster virus)	Mucosal vesicles and ulcers
HIV	Gingivitis
Measles (prodrome)	Koplik's spots (red spots in buccal mucosa)

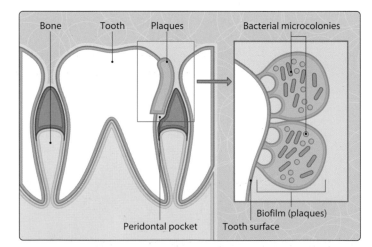

Fig. 3.46.1 Dental plaques and biofilms.

IgA) inhibits bacterial growth. Saliva also contains bicarbonate, which can buffer acidic pH, and its physical flow helps to remove microorganisms from the tooth surface. The regular brushing of teeth assists in the removal of plaques and foodstuff and combined with toothpaste (sodium lauryl sulphate) or mouth-washes (e.g. chlorhexidine) augments the killing of the bacteria. **Fluoride** (supplemented in toothpaste, water or food) inhibits bacterial metabolism and strengthens the tooth by incorporation into the enamel.

Periodontal disease

Periodontal (gum) disease is an infection of the supporting tissue of the teeth and often develops as a result of poor oral hygiene or immunosuppression. **Gingivitis** is a mild form of periodontal disease caused by bacterial plaques. The gum becomes red, inflamed and swollen and bleeds easily but with little discomfort. If left untreated, gingivitis can progress to **periodontitis**. This is an inflammatory condition caused by plaques extending along the tooth and below the gum line, forming periodontal pockets. A number of anaerobic bacteria (e.g. *Porphyromonas*, *Fusobacterium* spp.) colonize these pockets and produce a proteolytic and alkaline pH environment. This results in destruction of the gum tissue and even bone. **Complications** are loose teeth or loss of teeth and abscesses.

Although most gingivitis is caused by bacteria, viruses such as HIV or herpes are also known to cause periodontal disease.

Vincent's angina is a very severe form of gingivitis, also known as acute necrotizing ulcerative gingivitis. Patients present with fever, extremely bad breath (**halitosis**) and bleeding gums caused by a mixture of bacteria such as *Fusobacterium* spp. and *Borellia vincentii*, which can be treated with antibiotics (e.g. metronidazole or penicillin). This condition (also known as 'trench mouth') was particularly common in the First World War.

Prevention

Plaque control, treatment of existing gingivitis and periodontitis as well as good oral health (regular tooth brushing, flossing, descaling) are key components for the prevention of periodontal disease.

Mouth ulcers

Mouth ulcers are painful localized erosions of the oral mucosa. This is a common condition and may have a number of causes (e.g. trauma, stress, vitamin deficiencies, other diseases such as inflammatory bowel disease, oral cancer, immune disorders). Infectious causes include herpes simplex virus (relatively common, in particularly in immunocompromised patients), which can be treated with aciclovir. *Candida* spp. may cause ulcers particularly in those with HIV infection or who have other forms of immunosuppression and after a course of antibiotics; it can be treated with antifungal agents (e.g. nystatin or fluconazole).

Oral bacteria causing systemic infections

Endocarditis may develop as a consequence of poor dental hygiene or after mechanical manipulations such as descaling of teeth. Oral bacteria (typically *S. mutans*) can enter the bloodstream for a short period (transient bacteraemia) and settle on heart valves, causing infective endocarditis.

Lemierres's syndrome (necrobacillosis) is an infective syndrome that classically affects young people, who present with a sudden onset of fever and sore throat followed by jugular vein thrombosis and metastatic (lung) abscesses. The condition is mainly caused by *Fusobacterium necrophorum* and is treatable with antibiotics (e.g. penicillins, cephalosporins or metronidazole).

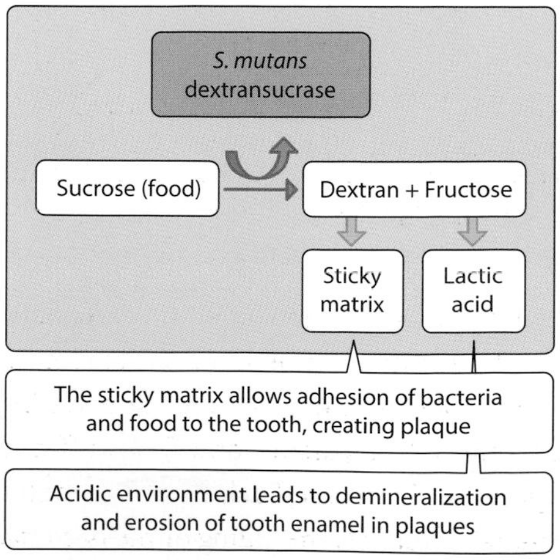

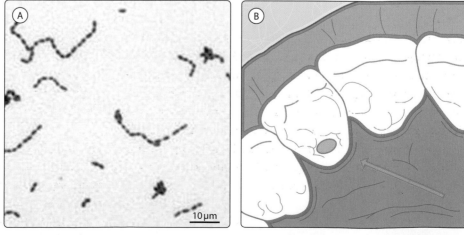

Fig. 3.46.2 Pathogenesis of dental decay.

Fig. 3.46.3 Dental caries. A. Gram stain of *Streptococcus mutans*, a cause of dental caries; B. caries in a tooth.

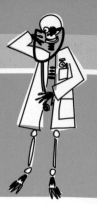

Appendix

Table A.1 DEFECTS IN IMMUNITY AND INFECTION

| | | Innate immunity | | Adaptive immunity | |
	Physical defences	Complement	Phagocytes	Humoral immunity (antibodies)	Cellular immunity
Main class attacked	Bacteria	Bacteria	Bacteria/fungi	Bacteria	Intracellular pathogens
Skin pathogens	*Staphylococcus aureus, Streptococcus* spp.	*Neisseria,* spp., *Haemophilus influenzae, Streptococcus pneumoniae, S. aureus*	*S. aureus, S. pneumoniae,* Gram-negative organisms	Enteroviruses, rotavirus, *S. aureus*	All viruses, especially herpesviruses, adenoviruses
Respiratory pathogens	Respiratory viruses, *S. pneumoniae, H. influenzae, Moraxella catarrhalis*		*Aspergillus, Candida* spp.	*S. pneumoniae, H. influenzae, Salmonella* spp., *Campylobacter* sp.	*Mycobacterium, Listeria, Salmonella, Legionella, Nocardia* spp.
Gastrointestinal pathogens	*Salmonella, Campylobacter,* Gram-negative organisms, anaerobes			*Giardia lamblia*	*Candida,* Aspergillus, *Cryptococcus, Pneumocystis* spp.
Urinary pathogens	*Escherichia coli,* Gram-negative organisms				*Toxoplasma, Cryptosporidium, Strongyloides* spp.
Genital pathogens	Anaerobes (bacterial vaginosis), *Candida* spp.				

Table A.2 NEWLY EMERGING PATHOGENS AND DISEASES

Year	Pathogen	Disease
1973	Rotavirus	Infantile diarrhoea
1975	Parvovirus B19	Aplastic crisis; fetal loss
1976	*Cryptosporidium*	Acute and chronic diarrhoea
1977	Ebola virus	Haemorrhagic fever
1977	*Legionella pneumophila*	Legionnaire's disease
1977	Hantaan virus	Haemorrhagic fever and renal syndrome
1977	*Campylobacter jejuni*	Diarrhoea
1980	Human T lymphotropic virus 1 (HTLV-1)	T cell lymphoma
1981	*Staphylococcus aureus* producing toxic shock syndrome toxin 1 (TSST-1)	Toxic shock syndrome
1982	*Escherichia coli* O157:H7	Haemorrhagic colitis; haemolytic uraemic syndrome
1982	Human T lymphotropic virus 2 (HTLV-2)	Hairy cell leukaemia
1982	*Borrelia burgdorferi* and related species	Lyme disease
1983	Human immunodeficiency virus (HIV)	Acquired immunodeficiency syndrome (AIDS)
1983	*Helicobacter pylori*	Peptic ulcer disease; gastric carcinoma
1984	*Haemophilus influenzae* bio. Aegyptius	Brazilian purpuric fever
1985	*Enterocytozoon bieneusi*	Persistent diarrhoea
1986	*Cyclospora cayetanensis*	Persistent diarrhoea
1986	HIV-2	AIDS
1988	Human herpesvirus 6 (HHV6)	Roseola subitum
1988	Hepatitis E	Enterally transmitted hepatitis
1989	Hepatitis C	Parenterally transmitted hepatitis
1989	*Ehrlichia chafeensis*	Human ehrlichiosis
1991	Guanarito virus	Venezuelan haemorrhagic fever
1991	*Encephalitozoon hellem*	Conjunctivitis, disseminated disease
1991	New species of *Babesia*	Atypical babesiosis
1991	*Tropheryma whippelii*	Whipple's disease
1992	*Vibrio cholerae* O139	Cholera
1992	*Bartonella henselae*	Cat scratch fever; bacillary angiomatosis
1993	Sin Nombre virus	Adult respiratory distress syndrome
1994	Sabia virus	Brazilian haemorrhagic fever
1995	Human herpes virus 8 (HHV8)	Kaposi's sarcoma in AIDS
1996	Bovine spongiform encephalopathy prion	Variant Creutzfeldt–Jacob disease
2001	Metapneumovirus	Bronchiolitis
2002	Severe acute respiratory syndrome coronavirus (SARS)	Fever, cough, flu-like illness with pneumonia

Table A.3 NOTIFIABLE INFECTIOUS DISEASES IN THE UK

In the UK, many infections are notifiable by law to the 'consultant in communicable diseases control' or other appropriate officer	
Disease	**Note**
Acute encephalitis	Not Scotland
Anthrax	
Chickenpox	Not England and Wales
Cholera	
Diphtheria	
Dysentery	
Food poisoning	Also suspected, in England and Wales
Gastroenteritis	If under 2 years of age, Northern Ireland only
Lassa fever	Separate category in England and Wales only
Legionellosis	Not England and Wales
Leprosy	Not Northern Ireland
Leptospirosis	
Malaria	
Measles	
Meningitis	'Acute' only in Northern Ireland
Meningococcal septicaemia without meningitis	Only England and Wales
Mumps	
Ophthalmia neonatorum	Only England and Wales
Paratyphoid fever	
Plague	
Poliomyelitis	
Puerperal fever	Scotland only
Rabies	
Relapsing fever	
Rubella	
Scarlet fever	Not Scotland
Smallpox	
Tetanus	Not Scotland
Tuberculosis	Not Scotland
Typhoid fever	Not Scotland
Typhus	
Viral haemorrhagic fever	
Viral hepatitis	
Whooping cough	
Yellow fever	Not Scotland

Table A.4 VACCINES AVAILABLE IN THE UK

Vaccine	Preparation	Additional comments
Diphtheria	Toxoid	UK immunization schedule
Tetanus	Toxoid	UK immunization schedule; postexposure prophylaxis
Pertussis	Whole cell killed	UK immunization schedule; acellular vaccines (pertussis toxin and haemagglutinin) becoming available
Haemophilus influenzae b	Capsular polysaccharide (conjugated)	UK immunization schedule; used in asplenic patients
Polio	Live attenuated	UK immunization schedule: oral (Sabin) in UK; inactivated injectable (Salk) also available
Measles	Live attenuated	UK immunization schedule
Mumps	Live attenuated	UK immunization schedule
Rubella	Live attenuated	UK immunization schedule; women of child-bearing age with no evidence of immunity
BCG	Live attenuated	UK immunization schedule
Anthrax	Toxin (enriched)	Only if risk of occupational exposure
Cholera		Unavailable in the UK; no longer recommended by the World Health Organization
Hepatitis A	Inactivated	Travellers to endemic area; outbreaks; occupational risk; haemophiliacs and those with liver disease
Hepatitis B	Single protein	Neonates of positive mother; occupational risk; lifestyle; postexposure prophylaxis
Influenza	Inactivated purified	Chronic respiratory disease; heart disease; renal failure; diabetes; immunosuppressed
Japanese encephalitis	Inactivated	Travellers to endemic area (unlicensed in UK; 'named patient basis' only)
Meningococcal (groups A & C)	Purified polysaccharide	Travellers to endemic area; outbreaks; postexposure prophylaxis; asplenic patients
	Conjugated vaccine (MenC)	Age < 25 years and those who may be at elevated risk from meningococcal infection
Pneumococcal	Purified polysaccharide	As for influenza *plus* asplenic patients
	Conjugate vaccine	For children
Rabies	Inactivated	Occupational risk; postexposure prophylaxis
Tick-borne encephalitis	Inactivated	Travellers to endemic area (unlicensed in UK; 'named patient basis' only)
Typhoid	Whole cell killed	Polysaccharide (Vi) and oral (Ty21a) vaccines now available: travellers to endemic area; occupational risk
Varicella zoster	Live attenuated	Immunocompromised (unlicensed in UK; 'named patient basis' only)
Yellow fever	Live attenuated	Travellers (to endemic area or if vaccination certificate required for entry)

Table A.5 STERILIZATION METHODS

Method	Example	Mode of action	Application
Dry heat	Heating in a flame: hot air oven at 160–180°C for 1 h; incineration at > 1000°C	Direct oxidation	Inoculating loops; metal instruments and glassware; disposal of infectious waste
Moist heat	Autoclaving: 121°C for 15 min or 134°C for 3 min	Protein denaturation	Preparation of surgical instruments and dressings; production of laboratory culture media and reagents; disposal of infectious waste
	Steaming: 100°C for 5 min on 3 consecutive days (Tyndallization)		Named after its originator: in a suitable liquid, spores will germinate on cooling and are then killed by the next day's steaming (the third heating is for extra security)
Irradiation	Cobalt-60 gamma irradiation	Damage of DNA through free-radical formation	Heat-labile items such as plastic syringes, needles and other small single-use items
Chemical	Ethylene oxide gas	Alkylating agents causing protein and nucleic acid damage	Toxic and potentially explosive; used for items that cannot withstand autoclaving (e.g. heart valves)
	Formaldehyde gas		Toxic and irritant; decontamination of microbiology laboratory rooms and safety cabinets
	Peracetic acid		Toxic and irritant; decontamination of laboratory equipment and instruments (e.g. endoscopes)
	Hydrogen peroxide gas plasma	Microwave frequency produces free radicals	Safe; decontamination of heat labile (dry) items
Filtration	Passing solutions through a defined pore-sized membrane (e.g. 0.2–0.45 μm)	Physical removal of microbes	Preparation of laboratory culture media, reagents and some pharmaceutical products

Table A.6 COMMONLY USED ABBREVIATIONS

As with all branches of medicine, abbreviations are routinely used in medical microbiology where they provide a convenient 'shorthand' for describing laboratory and clinical findings. However, abbreviations should be used cautiously as they may be employed in another branch of medicine to describe a totally different test or clinical finding. Below is a list of some common medical microbiology abbreviations.

AAFB	acid–alcohol-fast bacilli
AFB	acid-fast bacilli
AHG	anti-human globulin (antibodies, serum)
ASO	antistreptolysin O
ATS	anti-tetanus serum
BCG	Bacille Calmette–Guérin
C1, C2, etc.	complement components
CFT	complement fixation test
CFU	colony-forming unit
CIE	countercurrent immunoelectrophoresis
CJD	Creutzfeldt–Jakob disease
CMV	cytomegalovirus
CPE	cytopathic effect
CSF	cerebrospinal fluid
CSU	catheter specimen of urine
CTL	cytotoxic T lymphocyte
DEAFF	detection of early antigen fluorescent foci (used for diagnosis of CMV)
DPT	diphtheria, pertussis, tetanus combined (triple) vaccine
EBV	Epstein–Barr virus
ECHO	enteric cytopathic human orphan (viruses)
ELISA	enzyme-linked immunosorbent assay
EMU	early morning urine (specimen of)
EPEC	enteropathogenic *Escherichia coli*
ETEC	enterotoxigenic *Escherichia coli*
Fab, Fc	antibody-binding (ab) and complement-binding (c) parts of immunoglobulin molecule
FTA	fluorescent treponemal antibody (test)
GALT	gut-associated lymphoid tissue
GC	gonococcus
GCFT	guanidine + cytosine mol% content of DNA
GLC	gas–liquid chromatography
HAI	haemagglutination inhibition (test)
HBsAg etc.	antigenic components of hepatitis B virus
Hib	*Haemophilus influenzae* type b
HIV	human immunodeficiency virus
HPV	human papilloma virus
HSV	herpes simplex virus
HTLV	human T cell lymphotropic virus
HUS	haemolytic uraemic syndrome

Continued

Table A.6 COMMONLY USED ABBREVIATIONS—cont'd

HVS	high vaginal swab
ID	infective dose
IFN	interferon
IgA, IgE, etc.	immunoglobulins of classes, A, E, etc.
IL	interleukin
IM	intramuscular
INAH	isonicotinic acid hydrazide isoniazid
IPV	inactivated polio vaccine
i.v. or IV	intravenous
K	capsular or envelope (antigens, antibodies)
LCR	ligase chain reaction
LD_{50}	dose lethal to 50% of a group of experimental animals
LF	lactose fermenter
LGV	lymphogranuloma venereum
LPS	lipopolysaccharide
LRTI	lower respiratory tract infection
LT	heat-labile toxin (of *Escherichia coli*)
Mab	monoclonal antibody
MBC	minimal bactericidal concentration
MIC	minimal inhibitory concentration
MIC_{90}	concentration that inhibits 90% of a group of bacterial strains
MIF	macrophage migration-inhibiting factor
MLD	minimum lethal dose (of a drug or microbial preparation)
MMR	measles, mumps, rubella (vaccine)
MRSA	methicillin-resistant (multiresistant) *Staphylococcus aureus*
MSU	midstream urine (specimen of)
NGU	non-gonococcal urethritis
NLF	non-lactose fermenter
NK	natural killer (cell)
NSU	non-specific urethritis
NSV	non-specific vaginitis (anaerobic vaginosis)
OPV	oral polio vaccine
PABA	*p*-aminobenzoic acid
PCR	polymerase chain reaction
pfu	plaque-forming unit
PGU	post-gonococcal urethritis
PMC	pseudomembranous colitis
PPD	purified protein derivative (of old tuberculin)
PUO	pyrexia of unknown origin
RIA	radioimmunoassay
RNA	ribonucleic acid

Table A.6 COMMONLY USED ABBREVIATIONS—cont'd

RSV	respiratory syncytial virus
SDD	selective decontamination of the digestive tract
SPEAR	specific parenteral and enteral antiseptic regimen
sp.	species (plural spp.)
STD/STI	sexually transmitted disease/infection
TAB (TABC)	typhoid + paratyphoids A and B (and C) vaccine
TB	tubercle bacilli (used to denote tuberculosis)
TCID	tissue culture infective dose
TNF	tumour necrosis factor
TORCH	toxoplasma, rubella virus, cytomegalovirus, herpes simplex virus (acronym for four infectious agents that must be considered in congenital infections)
TPHA	*Treponema pallidum* haemagglutination (test)
TPI	*Treponema pallidum* immobilization (test)
TRIC	trachoma and inclusion conjunctivitis (agents)
TT	(1) tetanus toxoid; (2) tuberculin tested (cattle)
URTI	upper respiratory tract infection
UTI	urinary tract infection
VDRL	Venereal Diseases Research Laboratory (test)
Vi	virulence (antigen of *Salmonella typhi*, etc.)
VRE	vancomycin-resistant enterococci
VT	vero cell cytotoxin (of *Escherichia coli*)
VTEC	verotoxin-producing *Escherichia coli*
VZV	varicella zoster (virus)
WR	Wassermann reaction
ZN	Ziehl–Neelsen (staining method used to detect mycobacteria)

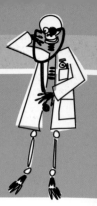

Further reading

This short book cannot fully do justice to the subject of infection. Most general medical textbooks have much more detail on the organisms, and review articles in medical and scientific journals will provide students with up-to-date comprehensive information on important infectious topics. There are also some specialist texts which can be 'dipped into' as supplemental reading for specific topics of interest.

Heyman DL (ed.) (1995) Control of communicable diseases, 18th edn. American Public Health Association, Washington, DC

Department of Health (1996) Immunisation against infectious disease. HMSO, London

Fraise A, Bradley C (eds) (2009) Ayliffe's control of health care associated infections. A practical handbook, 5th edn. Arnold, London

Greenwood D, Slack R, Peutherer J (eds) (2003) Medical microbiology, 16th edn. Churchill Livingstone, Edinburgh

Greenwood D, Finch R, Davey P, Wilcox M (eds) (2006) Antimicrobial chemotherapy, 5th edn. Oxford University Press, Oxford

Mandell GL, Bennett JE, Dolin R (eds) (2005) Principles and practice of infectious disease, 6th edn. Churchill Livingstone, New York

Mims C, Dimmock N, Nash A, Stephen J (2001) Mims' pathogenesis of infectious disease, 5th edn. Academic Press, London

Glossary

acid-fast bacteria retaining initial stain and difficult to decolorize with acid alcohol

aerobe any oxygen-requiring organism; cf. anaerobe

aetiology the study of the cause of a disease

agar a dried polysaccharide extract of seaweed used as a solidifying agent in microbiological media

anaerobe an organism that grows in the absence of molecular oxygen; cf. aerobe

antagonism the killing, injury or inhibition of growth of one species of microorganism by another when one organism adversely affects the environment of the other

antibiotic a substance of microbial origin that has antimicrobial activity

antimicrobial agent any chemical or biological agent that destroys or inhibits growth of microorganisms

antiseptic a disinfectant that can be applied to the skin to prevent or stop growth of microorganisms

antitoxin an antibody capable of uniting with and neutralizing a specific toxin

arthropod an invertebrate with jointed legs, e.g. an insect or a crustacean

asepsis a condition in which harmful microorganisms are absent

aseptic technique precautionary measures taken to prevent contamination

asymptomatic exhibiting no symptoms

attenuation weakening, reduction in virulence

autoclave an apparatus using steam under pressure for sterilization

bacillus any rod-shaped bacterium

bacteraemia bacteria in the bloodstream

bactericide an agent that destroys bacteria

bacteriophage a virus that infects bacteria and causes lysis of bacterial cells

bacteriostasis inhibition of growth and reproduction of bacteria without killing them

bacterium (pl. bacteria) diverse and ubiquitous prokaryotic single-celled microorganism

bacteriuria excretion of bacteria in urine

beta haemolysis a colourless, defined zone of haemolysis surrounding certain bacterial colonies growing on blood agar

capsule an envelope or slime layer surrounding the cell wall of certain microorganisms

carrier a person in apparently good health who harbours a pathogenic microorganism

chancre the primary ulcerative lesion in syphilis

chemotaxis movement of an organism in response to a chemical stimulus

chemotherapy treatment of disease by the use of chemicals

cilium (pl. cilia) a hair-like appendage on certain cells

clone a population of cells descended from a single cell

coagulase an enzyme produced by pathogenic staphylococci that causes coagulation of blood plasma

coccus a spherical bacterium

colony a macroscopically visible growth of microorganisms on a solid culture medium

commensalism relationship between members of different species living in proximity in which one organism benefits from the association but the other is not affected

compromised host a person already weakened by debilitating disease

conjugation a mating process characterized by the temporary fusion of the mating partners and transfer of genes; conjugation occurs particularly in unicellular organisms

contamination entry of undesirable organisms into some material or object

culture population of microorganisms cultivated in a medium

decimal reduction time time required to reduce a viable microbial population by 90%, usually applied to heat or chemical disinfection

denature modification, by physical or chemical action, of the structure of an organic substance (e.g. protein) in order to alter some properties of the substance, such as solubility

dimorphism occurring in two forms

disease a state of impaired body function occurring as a response to infection, stress or other condition

disinfectant an agent that kills most, but not all, microorganisms

DNA polymerase an enzyme that synthesizes DNA by adding nucleotides in one direction

dysentery disease caused by infection of the lower intestine

endemic peculiar to or occurring constantly in a community

endogenous produced or originating from within

endotoxin toxin produced in an organism and liberated only when the organism disintegrates

enteric pertaining to the intestines

enteropathogen organism that causes intestinal disease

enterotoxin a toxin specific for cells of the intestine; it gives rise to symptoms of food poisoning

epidemic a sudden increase in the incidence of a disease, affecting large numbers of people over a wide area

epidemiology the study of the factors that influence the occurrence and distribution of disease in groups of individuals

ETEC enterotoxin-producing *Escherichia coli*, causing gastroenteritis

eukaryote a cell that possesses a definitive or true nucleus; cf. prokaryote

exogenous produced or originating from without

exospore a spore external to the vegetative cell

exotoxin a toxin excreted by a microorganism into the surrounding medium

F factor fertility or sex factor in the cytoplasm of 'male' bacterial cells

fibrinolysin a substance produced by haemolytic streptococci that can liquefy clotted blood plasma or fibrin clots; also called streptokinase

fimbria (pl. fimbriae) surface appendage composed of protein subunits; term is often used interchangeably with pilus (qv.) but is usually restricted to the short appendages that occur in greater numbers and are specialized for attachment to a host cell

fission an asexual process by which some microorganisms reproduce

flagellates one of the subphyla of the phylum Protozoa

flagellum (pl. flagella) whip-like appendage on cells used for locomotion

flora (microbial) the microorganisms present in a given situation, e.g. intestinal flora

fomite a non-food substance or surface that is a potential source of infection, e.g. clothing

fulminating infection a sudden, severe and rapidly progressing infectious disease

fungicide an agent that kills or destroys fungi

gamete a reproductive cell (sex cell) that fuses with another reproductive cell to form a zygote, which then develops into a new individual

gastroenteritis inflammation of the mucosa of the stomach and intestine

generation time the time interval necessary for a cell to divide

genotype the particular set of genes present in an organism and its cells; an organism's genetic constitution; cf. phenotype

genus (pl. genera) a group of very closely related species

germicide an agent capable of killing germs, usually pathogenic microorganisms

Gram stain a differential stain by which bacteria are classed as Gram positive or Gram negative based on the chemical and physical properties of their cell walls; these determine whether the cells retain or lose the primary stain (crystal violet) when subjected to treatment with a decolorizing agent

Gram-negative bacteria bacteria that appear red after being subjected to the Gram stain; a number are medically relevant, e.g. *Hemophilus influenzae*, *Klebsiella pneumoniae*, *Legionella pneumophila*, *Pseudomonas aeruginosa*, *Escherichia coli*, *Helicobacter pylori*, *Salmonella enteritidis*, *Salmonella typhi*

Gram-positive bacteria bacteria that appear blue or violet after being subjected to the Gram stain, e.g. streptococci, staphylococci, *Corynebacterium*, *Listeria*, *Bacillus*, *Clostridium* spp.

H antigen a type of antigen found in the flagella of certain bacteria

haemolysis the process of dissolving red blood cells

HEPA high-efficiency particulate filtered air; free from airborne particles inclusive pathogens

hospital-acquired infection (HAI) infection acquired during the hospital stay that was not incubating or present at the time of admission; also referred to as nosocomial disease

host an organism harbouring another as a parasite or infectious agent

ID infective dose; the number of microorganisms required to infect a host

ID$_{50}$ the dose (number of microorganisms) that will infect 50% of the experimental animals in a test series

incubation in microbiology, the subjecting of cultures of microorganisms to conditions (especially temperatures) favourable to their growth

infectious capable of producing disease in a susceptible host

inoculation the artificial introduction of microorganisms or substances into the body or into a culture medium

inoculum the substance, containing microorganisms or other material, that is introduced in inoculation

in vitro literally 'in glass' and pertaining to biological experiments performed in test tubes or other laboratory vessels; cf. in vivo

in vivo within the living organism; pertaining to laboratory testing of agents within living organisms; cf. in vitro

Koch's postulates guidelines to prove that a disease is caused by a specific microorganism

LD$_{50}$ the dose (number of microorganisms) that will kill 50% of the animals in a test series

MBL mannose-binding lectin, a host protein that can opsonize pathogens or activate complement (was known as mannose-binding protein)

MIC minimal inhibitory concentration of an antimicrobial agent; the concentration at which bacteria just fail to grow

morphology the branch of biological science that deals with the study of the structure and form of living organisms

mycology the study of fungi

mycoplasma a group of bacteria composed of highly pleomorphic (many shaped) cells

mycosis a disease caused by fungi

mycotoxin any toxic substance produced by fungi

nosocomial disease describing or pertaining to disease acquired in the hospital that was not incubating or present at the time of admission; often now referred to as hospital-acquired infection (HAI)

oedema excessive accumulation of fluid in body tissue

opportunistic microorganism a microorganism that exists as part of the normal microbiota (flora) but becomes pathogenic when transferred from the normal habitat into other areas of the host or when host resistance is lowered

pandemic an epidemic of infectious disease that is spreading through human populations across a large region, e.g. a continent or worldwide

parasite an organism that derives its nourishment from a living plant or animal host; a parasite does not necessarily cause disease

parasitism the relationship of a parasite to its host

parenteral by some route other than via the intestinal tract

pasteurization the process of heating liquid food or beverage at a controlled temperature to enhance the keeping quality and destroy microorganisms

pathogen an organism capable of producing disease

peritrichous having flagella around the entire surface of the cell

phage see bacteriophage

phage typing identifying a pathogenic bacterium by the pattern of lysis caused by different phage types

phenotype the observable characteristics of an organism; cf. genotype

phylogeny the evolutionary or ancestral history of organisms

phylum (pl. phyla) a taxon consisting of a group of related classes

pilus (pl. pili) surface appendage responsible for linking the interiors of two bacteria for transmission of genetic material (conjugation); there are usually one or two per cell; cf. fimbria

potable suitable for drinking

prokaryote a type of cell in which the nuclear substance is not enclosed within a membrane, e.g. a bacterium; cf. eukaryote

prophylaxis preventive treatment for protection against disease

protist a microorganism in the kingdom Protista

protozoan (pl. protozoa) single-celled eukaryotic microorganism

protozoology the study of protozoa

pseudopodium a temporary projection of the protoplast of an amoeboid cell in which cytoplasm flows during extension and withdrawal

resistance-transfer factor (R) a factor that confers on microorganisms resistance to a number of antibiotics

pyuria the presence of white blood cells in urine

rickettsia obligate intracellular bacteria of arthropods, many types of which are pathogenic for humans and other mammals

sanitizer an agent that reduces the microbial flora in materials or on such articles as eating utensils to levels judged safe by public health authorities

saprophyte an organism living on dead organic matter

schizogony asexual reproduction by multiple fission of a trophozoite (a vegetative protozoan)

schizont a stage in the asexual life cycle of the malaria parasites

septicaemia a systemic disease caused by the invasion and multiplication of pathogenic microorganisms in the bloodstream

sequela (pl. sequelae) a complication following a disease

sequestrum (pl. sequestra) necrotic bone tissue in osteomyelitis

species a single kind of microorganism; a subdivision of a genus; abbreviation sp. (pl. spp.)

spirochaete a spiral form of bacterium; most are parasitic

spore a resistant body formed by certain microorganisms; a resistant resting cell; a primitive unicellular dormant body

sporicide an agent that kills spores

sporozoite a motile infective stage of certain sporozoans, resulting from sexual reproduction, that gives rise to an asexual cycle in a new host

sterile free of living organisms

sterilization the process of making sterile by killing all forms of life

stock cultures known species of microorganisms maintained in the laboratory for various tests and studies

strain a pure culture of microorganisms composed of the descendants of a single isolation

streptococci members of the genus *Streptococcus*; cocci divide in such a way that chains of cells are formed

susceptibility the state of being open to disease; specifically capability of being infected, lack of immunity

symbiosis the living together of two or more organisms; microbial association

syndrome a group of signs and symptoms that characterizes a disease

systematics the science of animal, plant and microbial classification

taxis movement away from or towards a chemical substance or physical condition

taxonomy the science of classification of organisms, usually based on natural relationships

teichoic acid a cell wall constituent unique to prokaryotes

thermolabile destroyed by heat at temperatures below 100°C

thermostable resistant to temperatures of 100°C

tissue culture a growth of tissue cells in vitro in a laboratory medium

topical application application to a localized area

toxin a poisonous substance elaborated by an organism, such as a bacterial toxin

trophozoite the vegetative form of a protozoan

tuberculin an extract of *Mycobacterium* bacillus capable of eliciting an inflammatory reaction in an animal body that has been sensitized by the presence of living or dead tubercle bacilli; used in a skin test (Mantoux) for tuberculosis

vaccination inoculation with a biological preparation (a vaccine) to produce immunity

vaccine a suspension of disease-producing microorganisms modified by killing or attenuation so that they will not cause disease and can stimulate the formation of antibodies upon inoculation

vector an agent, such as an insect, capable of mechanically or biologically transferring a pathogen from one organism to another

vegetative stage the stage of active growth, as opposed to the resting or spore stages

viable capable of living, growing and developing; alive

viraemia the presence of virus in the blood

viricide an agent that kills viruses

virology the study of viruses

virulence the capacity of a microorganism to produce disease; pathogenicity

virus acellular microorganisms smaller than bacteria with a simple organization and possessing either DNA or RNA; they cannot replicate independently of host cells so are obligate intracellular parasites

VTEC verotoxin-producing *Escherichia coli*, usually serotype O157, causing colitis

yeast a kind of fungus that is unicellular and not characterized by typical mycelia

zoonosis disease transmitted to humans from animals

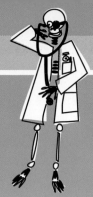

Index